UNDERSTANDING AND
MANAGEMENT OF NAUSEA
AND VOMITING

UNDERSTANDING AND MANAGEMENT OF NAUSEA AND VOMITING

Jan Hawthorn
BSc, PhD

Blackwell
Science

© 1995 by Jan Hawthorn
Blackwell Science Ltd
Editorial Offices:
Osney Mead, Oxford OX2 0EL
25 John Street, London WC1N 2BL
23 Ainslie Place, Edinburgh EH3 6AJ
238 Main Street, Cambridge
  Massachusetts 02142, USA
54 University Street, Carlton
  Victoria 3053, Australia

Other Editorial Offices:
Arnette Blackwell SA
1, rue de Lille, 75007 Paris
France

Blackwell Wissenshafts-Verlag GmbH
Kurfürstendamm 57
10707 Berlin, Germany

Blackwell MZV
Feldgasse 13, A-1238 Wien
Austria

First published 1995

Typeset by DP Photosetting,
Aylesbury, Bucks
Printed and bound in Great Britain by
Hartnolls Ltd, Bodmin, Cornwall

DISTRIBUTORS

Marston Book Services Ltd
PO Box 87
Oxford OX2 0DT
(*Orders:* Tel: 01865 791155
         Fax: 01865 791927
         Telex: 837515)

USA
Blackwell Science, Inc.
238 Main Street
Cambridge, MA 02142
(*Orders:* Tel: 800 759-6102
         617 876-7000)

Canada
Times Mirror Professional
  Publishing Ltd
130 Flaska Drive
Markham, Ontario L6G 1B8
(*Orders:* Tel: 800 268-4178
         Fax: 416 470-6739)

Australia
Blackwell Science Pty Ltd
54 University Street
Carlton, Victoria 3053
(*Orders:* Tel: 03 347-5552)

A catalogue record for this title
is available from the British Library

ISBN 0–632–03819–5

Library of Congress
Cataloging-in-Publication Data

Hawthorn, Jan.
    Understanding and management
of nausea and vomiting/Jan
Hawthorn.
        p.   cm.
    Includes bibliographical
references and index.
    ISBN 0–632–03819–5
    1. Nausea.   2. Vomiting.
3. Nausea–Nursing.   4. Vomiting–
Nursing.   I. Title.
    [DNLM: 1. Nausea–nursing.
2. Vomiting–nursing.
3. Antiemetics–nurses' instruction.
WY 156.5 H399u 1994]
RB150.N38H39   1994
616'.047–dc20
DNLM/DLC
for Library of Congress   94-31283
                                CIP

CONTENTS

CONTRIBUTORS

A.C.M. Eberhardie, TD, MSc, RGN, RNT, MHSM is Reader in Neuroscience Nursing at Kingston and St. George's NHS College of Health Studies, London.

A. Phylip Pritchard, BA, RGN, RMN is European Officer at the Royal College of Nursing, London.

Kathy Redmond, MSc, RGN, Cert. Onc., is Lecturer in the Department of Nursing Studies, University College, Dublin.

Pat Webb, RGN, RCNT, RNT, Dip.Soc.Res., is Lecturer in Palliative Care at Trinity Hospice, London.

Saffron Whitehead, BSc, PhD, is Senior Lecturer in the Department of Physiology, St. George's Hospital Medical School, London.

ACKNOWLEDGEMENTS

The idea of writing a book for nurses about nausea and vomiting was not entirely mine. It had evolved from the joint collaboration of members of the International Society of Nurses in Cancer Care and Glaxo, who wanted to produce a learning package written specifically for cancer nurses. I was invited to write the package and through that project I developed a greater understanding of the whole science as well as art of nursing and made some very valuable friends.

The package was adapted in a similar venture for surgical nurses, to help in the management of postoperative nausea and vomiting where once again I received valuable and enthusiastic support.

With encouragement from many people involved in these two projects, I have now written this book which covers the problems of nausea and vomiting in a variety of situations.

This book could not have been written without the enthusiastic support and contributions of several people. I am especially grateful to the reviewers, who also contributed much advice and information: Phylip Pritchard, Kathy Redmond, Pat Webb, Saffron Whitehead and Chris Eberhardie and to Nora Lawson and Sue Hutchinson who gave me much help and valuable information. I am indebted to Paul Andrews whose advice and discussions have been invaluable over the years.

I have also learned much from other nurses notably; Andrea Hill, Gertrud Grahn, Gill Chadwick, Virginia Gumley, Mark Darley, Moya Berli, Ria Dubbelman, Margaret Fitch, Anne Hilton, Kirsten Kopp and Inge Olsen. My sincere thanks to them all.

My special thanks go to Graham Baker who not only was instrumental in bringing the initial projects to fruition but whose kindness and generosity in allowing me to reproduce some of the original teaching package material has helped greatly.

Lastly I would like to acknowledge my debt to the late Robert Tiffany who contributed so much enthusiasm to the initial project and whose humour, warmth and compassion for cancer patients was an inspiration.

CHAPTER 1:
INTRODUCTION

At some point in their careers, all nurses will be called upon to care for patients suffering from nausea and/or vomiting. The severity of nausea and vomiting can cover a wide spectrum ranging from the occasional, unpleasant, but trivial event – at least in medical terms – to the extremely distressing and debilitating prolonged nausea and vomiting associated with some types of cancer therapy. Nausea and vomiting may simply be the result of overindulgence which is quickly resolved once the patient has vomited or may be significant clinical symptoms pointing to a more serious underlying condition. Nurses will also encounter nausea and vomiting in expectant mothers, on paediatric wards and when nursing surgical patients either in the recovery room or on their return to the ward. Casualty nurses or general practice nurses may be confronted by a patient who is suffering from a sudden and serious bout of vomiting. This can be very alarming for a patient especially if there is blood in the vomitus.

It is essential, therefore, that nurses have some awareness of the importance of nausea and vomiting as symptoms, understand what causes nausea and vomiting and are well equipped to deal with them.

Unfortunately, nausea and vomiting are often neglected topics in nurse education. For example, a survey of cancer nurses in 1989 showed that nearly 80% of their training in how to manage nausea and vomiting was 'on-the-job' and the nurses' evaluation of the quality of training was only slightly better than 'inadequately covered' (Pritchard & Speechley, 1990). This is in spite of the fact that cancer treatment, especially chemotherapy, has long been known to be associated with prolonged nausea and vomiting. Even the general public have a perception that the worst aspect of their medical treatment for cancer will be the sickness. In a much quoted survey in 1983, 'being sick' and 'feeling sick' were rated as the first and second most distressing problems for cancer patients (Coates *et al.*, 1983).

A more recent article (anonymous) in 1993 in the *Nursing Times* reported on a survey of members of The Association of Theatre Nurses. When asked for their opinion on postoperative nausea and vomiting (PONV) 94% expressed concern over PONV. Nurses believed that PONV could lead to life-threatening complications, affected ward morale and the allocation of nursing time. PONV has also been reported as one of the most unpleasant aspects of the postoperative period for patients (Cronin *et al.*, 1973).

This book is written for nurses and aims to provide a text which covers the physiology of nausea and vomiting, the aetiology of different types of nausea and vomiting, the use of anti-emetic drugs, and other interventions, to control nausea and vomiting and the nursing strategies for caring for patients who are suffering from nausea and vomiting either because of illness or as a side-effect of treatment.

CHAPTER 2: THE PHYSIOLOGY OF NAUSEA AND VOMITING

2.1 Factors causing vomiting

Vomiting can be caused by a surprisingly diverse range of stimuli, (Table 2.1). What is fascinating, from a physiological point of view, is that some mechanism is triggered by this disparate group of events that results in the same end points – nausea and vomiting.

Vomiting clearly has a psychological component; many of the agents from the list below are external events perceived by higher brain centres and translated into the act of vomiting. The 'translation' of these events is poorly understood in physiological terms. Other stimuli, however, have more obvious physical or chemical actions; over-distension of the stomach or eating food that has 'gone off' and contains toxins produces physiological events that can be fairly well explained.

Table 2.1 Factors causing nausea and vomiting

overindulgence (in food or drink)	pyloric stenosis
	tumour lysis syndrome
pregnancy	diabetic gastroparesis
travel (motion)	labyrinthitis
foul smells	vestibular neuronitis
horrific sights	pancreatitis
radiation	uraemia
chemotherapy	some cancers
anxiety	Addison's disease
bacterial or viral infection	hypercalcaemia
(including contaminated food)	diabetic ketoacidosis
extreme pain	mesenteric ischaemia
intestinal obstruction	heart attack
squashed stomach syndrome	Reye's syndrome
opiate analgesics e.g. morphine	hepatitis
surgical procedures	some drugs e.g. levodopa, AZT
raised intercranial pressure	anaesthetic agents

2.2 Why do we vomit?

Vomiting is essentially a protective mechanism. In biological terms, an animal's main aim in life is survival. Eating something poisonous is potentially disastrous – threatening the survival of the species. The animal needs, therefore, a way of reversing its mistake – vomiting. Vomiting will remove the poison from the body and thus remove the danger.

Feeling sick (nausea) is related to this process. Eating a small amount of a poisonous substance, produces unpleasant sensations that cause the animal to stop eating. (Sometimes smelling something that is 'off' produces unpleasant nausea-like sensations that prevent the substance being eaten at all). When nausea occurs digestion is halted, which prevents the toxin being absorbed and moving further into the body. Vomiting then occurs to remove the offending material (see Davis *et al.*, 1986). This is a good explanation of why, as animals, we have a vomiting reflex but a lot of nausea and vomiting encountered in the everyday life is not performing a 'defensive' role. When viewed as a defence mechanism, however, some of the nausea and vomiting encountered in the clinical situation does not seem quite so bizarre. For example, cytotoxic therapy is, by design, poisonous (Gk. *cyto* = cell, *toxic* = poison). Radiation also kills cells. Attempts are made to limit the extent to which these therapies are toxic. For example, radiation is targeted or focused on certain areas of the body and cytotoxic drugs are chosen because they attack rapidly dividing cells and not all body tissue (although some cells such as hair follicles are more susceptible). Unfortunately, the body cannot appreciate this subtlety. It detects the presence of a toxic substance and adopts the only response available to remove it – vomiting. In the case of cancer therapy this response is futile, but it is not wholly inappropriate. A more detailed explanation of how cytotoxic drugs and radiation are thought to cause nausea and vomiting is given in Chapter 3.

Such rational explanations cannot be invoked to explain why motion or pregnancy should cause nausea and vomiting; neither condition is particularly harmful or undesirable (at least in biological terms). What is happening in these cases is not so well understood.

2.3 The process of nausea and vomiting

Nausea and vomiting may be divided into three phases:

- nausea
- retching and vomiting
- post-vomiting

2.4 Nausea

Nausea is a subjective sensation that is fairly difficult to describe. Most definitions of nausea usually relate it to vomiting – the majority of textbooks refer to nausea as 'a desire to vomit'. A useful definition is that nausea is 'an unpleasant, but not painful sensation associated with the back of the throat and the gut and giving rise to the feeling that vomiting is imminent.' (The word nauseating is also used colloquially to denote feelings of disgust or loathing.)

This linking of nausea with vomiting is in some ways unfortunate since many people regard nausea as synonymous with vomiting. This is clearly not the case for, although there is an obvious connection between the two events, nausea does not necessarily culminate in vomiting. Conversely vomiting can sometimes be sudden and unheralded by feelings of nausea. For some patients nausea may be the more distressing problem as it can be more prolonged and less easily controlled than vomiting. Nausea and vomiting should, therefore, be considered as separate phenomena. Different anti-emetic drugs or techniques may have different effects on nausea and on vomiting. Only half the problem has been addressed if vomiting is controlled but there is no relief from nausea.

What causes nausea?

The vagueness in defining nausea perhaps reflects a less than complete understanding of nausea. What is known is that nausea is associated with the gut and, usually, with changes in gut motility patterns. The normal stomach is constantly contracting and relaxing with a regular rhythm. Nausea disturbs this rhythm causing a slowing or even complete cessation of gastric motility (gastric stasis), a loss of gastric tone and the stomach can become quite flaccid. This decrease in gastric motility will stop further digestion of food and absorption of toxins. Duodenal motion is reversed and retroperistalsis will move the contents of the duodenum back up into the stomach ready for expulsion from the body (Akwari, 1983; Lee *et al.*, 1985). Before vomiting occurs there is a single large contraction of the small intestine, called the retrograde giant contraction or RGC, which propagates in a retrograde fashion towards the stomach (Davidson & Pilot, 1993).

Excessively fatty food can also have an effect on gastric motility and this may be why large amounts of very rich food (for example double cream) can make you feel sick. This change in gastric motility may be related to the degree of nausea. It is interesting to note that some gastrokinetic agents (agents which stimulate gastric motility), such as cisapride, have little direct anti-emetic activity but a surprising degree of anti-nausea activity (Creytens, 1984).

When nausea occurs secretion of gastric acid decreases and salivation increases. Both of these may be attempts by the body to reduce the damage the strong gastric acid could have on the oesophagus and mouth. (Saliva is alkaline and would, therefore, buffer the stomach contents which are at a pH of about 1–4).

It is noticeable that in patients with bulimia nervosa – who will often make themselves sick by putting their fingers down their own throat – erosion of the enamel on the back of their teeth occurs. Presumably this is because these individuals do not experience nausea before being sick and the changes in gastric acid and saliva do not have time to occur. The strong stomach acid, therefore, is more liable to harm their teeth.

When patients feel nauseous they usually appear pale, experience cold sweats, may have tachycardia and increased pulse rate, and feel cold or clammy. All these are signs of increased activity of the sympathetic nervous system. Just why this should occur is not known. The factors associated with nausea are summarized in Table 2.2.

The function of nausea is not known but it has been suggested that, in biological terms it is an aversive stimulus. That is, if something causes an animal to feel nauseous it will avoid that thing in the future.

Biochemical changes associated with nausea include decreased urine output, decreased glucose utilization, increased lactic dehydrogenase levels, decreased end tidal CO_2 production and increased blood pH. Plasma vasopressin levels are vastly increased (20–50, fold). This observation has not been explained, but the role of vasopressin has generated some

Table 2.2 Factors associated with nausea

- changes in gastric motility
- gastric relaxation
- retroperistalsis in the duodenum
- decreases in gastric acid secretion
- increased salivation
- pallor
- cold sweats
- tachycardia

interest as it is possibly a biochemical factor that could be measured to give an objective assessment of the degree of nausea.

Evaluating nausea Nausea is a subjective experience and, as such, can only be evaluated by the patient or by eliciting information from the patient. The experienced nurse, however, will be sensitive to changes in the patient's attitude and external cues which may signal discomfort. But even when such clues are present the nurse will still have to ask how the patient is feeling.

Usually the amount of nausea does not need to be evaluated, just establishing whether nausea is present or not is sufficient to determine treatment. However, for clinical trials assessing the efficacy of anti-emetics we need to be able to measure nausea to see if interventions are successful. The experience of nausea is recorded on a form by the patient, a nurse or some other observer. In the former case, the person conducting the survey must take time to explain and ensure that the patient understands the type of assessment being used. If an observer is completing the form the observer will need time to ask how the patient is feeling.

There are two main ways of recording nausea: using a semantic scale or using a visual analogue scale (VAS).

The semantic scale (or discrete scale) consists of words suggesting the degree of nausea. A typical scale would include the range: none – mild – moderate – severe. The patient is asked to assess the nausea in these terms at various times. Many researchers feel it is important not to have an odd number of variables as some patients will just opt for the mid-point without thinking about the options. An even number of choices means that no word is at the mid-point and they need to make a decision.

A VAS consists of a 10 cm line marked 'no nausea' at one end and something like 'extreme nausea' at the other. The line may be vertical, but is more commonly horizontal. Patients are asked to mark the point along the line which best represents their feelings. Examples of both types of scale are given in Figure 2.1.

Sometimes a coloured strip rather than a line is employed, but the principle remains the same. This is called an analogue continuous chromatic scale (ACCS). The strip is graded from a very pale colour at one end marked 'no nausea', which darkens to an intense shade of the same colour at the other end and is marked something like 'severe nausea' or 'worst nausea I have ever felt'. Patients use a vertical black line to mark the point which represents their feelings. The investigator then measures the distance from the origin – effectively converting this to an analogue scale. The analogue scales were originally devised for measuring pain.

While initially both analogue scales seem a good idea, in practice they are often beset with problems. Many patients find the concept hard to understand. Some forms are returned marked with 10 or 12 lines; sometimes marks are made elsewhere on the page that bear little relationship to the line;

NAUSEA (feeling sick)

Tick one box only for each day

DAY	1 Day of therapy	2	3	4	5
DATE					
NONE					
MILD					
MODERATE					
SEVERE					

(a)

No nausea ■━━━━━━━━━━━━━━━━━━━■ Worst nausea
I have ever felt

(b)

Figure 2.1 Examples of scales for measuring nausea. Nausea can be measured on a semantic or descriptive scale (a) or a visual analogue scale (b).

patients will often circle the wording at the end of the line. Even if the concept can be explained successfully different studies using a VAS cannot always be compared as patients will react differently depending on the wording at the end of the line or the way the line is drawn e.g. whether the line is divided into sections or is a continuous uninterrupted line (Figure 2.1).

A recent study has shown that there is a close correlation between results obtained within the same group of patients whether a VAS or an ACCS was used, which is perhaps not surprising as both scales are analysed in the same way. The correlation between these scales and a semantic scale was also good (Del Favero *et al.*, 1990). Interestingly, this study also showed that the quantity or total entity of nausea were better measurements to make rather than just the maximum intensity or the duration of nausea. The quantity is obtained by adding all the nausea scores (on either a semantic or analogue scale) over the entire period of the study. The limitations of each type of assessment are discussed in more detail by Del Favero and colleagues (Del Favero *et al.*, 1992; Tonato *et al.*, 1993).

Some researchers have devised their own scales for assessing nausea. These usually consist of measuring several parameters during the study (Rhodes *et al.*, 1984; Morrow, 1984a; Morrow, 1992). Such scales have been published but have not become widely adopted in anti-emetic research.

Another point worth thinking about when evaluating studies of nausea is when the patient is questioned. If a patient is feeling very nauseated when the time comes to fill in the questionnaire (or the nurse asks) then they will clearly rate their nausea as very bad. If, however the nausea has passed – the patient has had a cup of tea or a cheering visit – they may look back on the experience and decide that, on reflection, it really wasn't that bad. Similarly the very act of giving someone a scale to fill in may make them dwell on their feelings and actually evoke sensations of nausea.

It is a well established practice in clinical research not to use leading questions to elicit information about side-effects of treatment; just suggesting that a mild symptom like a headache is a possible side-effect often brings a positive response from the patient – sometimes just because the patient 'doesn't want to disappoint the investigator'. It could be argued that to present a scale to be completed is in itself a very leading question.

Until there is a universally agreed method of assessing nausea it will be difficult to compare different studies on the effects of anti-emetic regimens and the above limitations should be borne in mind.

2.5 Retching

Retching is the rhythmic movement that usually occurs in bursts immediately before vomiting. Sometimes called 'dry heaves', retching is essentially breathing in against a closed glottis. The respiratory muscles act exactly as they would during the taking of a deep breath. The external intercostal muscles, the whole of the diaphragm and the abdominal muscles contract together causing rhythmic decreases in intrathoracic pressure with concomitant increases in abdominal pressure (McCarthy & Borison, 1974). (Figure 2.2). Autoradiographic studies have shown that during each negative oscillation in intrathoracic pressure the gastric contents oscillate between stomach and oesophagus.

Immediately before vomiting the lower oesophagus shortens drawing the stomach up towards the diaphragm and possibly

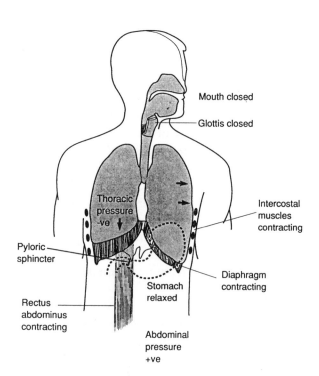

Figure 2.2 Retching. Retching is essentially breathing in against a closed glottis.

reducing the angle between the fundus and the oesophagus (the angle of His) (Lang, 1990). This facilitates the passage of the gastric contents when the stomach is compressed.

The function of retching is unknown but it has been suggested that perhaps retching moves the duodenal and stomach contents to an appropriate position for removal. The number of retches occurring may be related to the nature and quantity of the gastric contents at the time (Andrews *et al.*, 1990a).

Retching can occur without vomiting. Such episodes are usually quite unpleasant and stressful for patients who often find this more uncomfortable than actually vomiting. People will often say that they retch but cannot be sick because their stomach is empty. This may be true if the body can 'detect', during the retching episode, that the stomach is empty and assumes, therefore, there is no need to vomit.

2.6 Vomiting

Sometimes the term emesis is used instead of vomiting. They mean the same thing. Vomit is derived from the Latin *vomere* = to throw up, emesis comes from the Greek *emetikos* = to vomit. Sometimes emesis is used to encompass both nausea and vomiting.

Vomiting is the forceful expulsion of gastric contents through the mouth. This is achieved by the sudden, powerful contraction of the respiratory muscles and, at the same time, a relaxation of the upper oesophageal sphincter and the peri-oesophageal diaphragm. The major driving force for the expulsion of the gastric contents is the powerful contraction of the *rectus abdominis* and the external oblique muscles overlying the stomach (Figure 2.3). As mentioned previously the stomach becomes quite still and flaccid and vomiting is not due to contraction of the stomach.

Pressures in both the thorax and abdomen are positive whereas during retching thoracic pressure is negative. This demonstrates the powerful force of the contraction of the abdominal muscles. It is only when this force is transmitted to the thorax that vomiting occurs.

Measuring retching and vomiting

For clinical trials it may be necessary to measure retches and vomits. The easiest way to measure them is simply to count and usually observation is sufficient to distinguish between the two. If clinical trials of anti-emetics are being undertaken

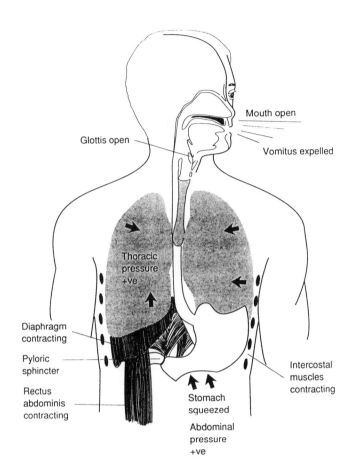

Mouth open

Glottis open

Vomitus expelled

Thoracic
pressure
+ve

Diaphragm
contracting

Pyloric
sphincter

Intercostal
muscles
contracting

Rectus
abdominis
contracting

Stomach
squeezed

Abdominal
pressure
+ve

Figure 2.3 Vomiting. Vomiting is the forceful expulsion of the gastric contents.

it is important to establish that the patient makes the distinction between retching and vomiting. If patients are being asked for information, or providing it by means of a diary card, then it must be quite clear what is defined as a retch and what as a vomit. A retch is often defined as 'a vomit unproductive of liquid'. It is clear from the preceding section that, in physiological terms, this is incorrect; they are different processes. However, at a practical level this is a useful working definition and the presence or absence of liquid can be used as a crude method to distinguish between the two if there is uncertainty. Where possible it is better for retching and vomiting to be assessed by an external observer since it will not be easy for someone undergoing the distressing experience of nausea and vomiting to count the number of events and note the time. In some circumstances the volume of vomitus may be measured. This is especially important where there is a high risk of dehydration and fluid balance is being closely monitored.

Even when such care is taken results are not always expressed the same way in clinical papers. The term 'emetic episode' is frequently employed and this can mean different things. Thus in different studies an emetic episode has been defined as:

- 1 vomit
- 1 retch or 1 vomit
- 1–5 retches
- 1–5 retches occurring within 5 minutes
- 1–5 retches or 1 vomit

The numbers of emetic episodes reported can vary considerably with these different methods of recording. As was discussed in the section on nausea, the time of questioning or assessment can be important. A study comparing concurrent with retrospective assessment of vomiting following gastric surgery showed that retrospective assessments exaggerated the frequency of vomiting (Stunkard *et al.*, 1985). If a patient is receiving anti-emetic medication that causes sedation or amnesia they will not be able to recall events accurately (Tonato *et al.*, 1993).

2.7 Post-vomiting phase

Vomiting is followed by lethargy and pronounced muscular weakness. Some patients find that their legs tremble and can no longer support them. If not in bed, the patient will probably need to sit down. The nature of this weakness is poorly understood. While vomiting is metabolically expensive and uses up considerable energy, this does not explain weakness of such severity. Sometimes patients also feel cold and shivery or experience muscular aches or pains.

At this point the patient may start to recover and gradually feel better or the whole cycle of events can be repeated. Nausea will increase and retching will occur followed by another vomit. Such bouts of repeated nausea and vomiting can last for several hours or, in the case of chemotherapy, for days or weeks.

2.8 Problems associated with nausea and vomiting

Prolonged nausea and vomiting is very debilitating, having a variety of consequences of varying severity (Table 2.3). Patients stop eating which in turn leads to weight loss and malnutrition – this can be inadequate calorie intake or inadequate intake of specific nutrients. Poor nutrition delays wound healing after surgery or recovery of damaged tissue after chemotherapy or radiotherapy.

Fluid loss can result in dehydration, hypotension and, in severe cases, mental confusion. Dehydration can also increase the nephrotoxicity of some drugs, especially cytotoxic drugs and to a lesser extent antibiotics. Care must be taken to ensure patients are well hydrated if they are receiving chemotherapy, especially in the case of cisplatin and aminoglycosides.

Electrolyte imbalance can occur, severe instances giving rise to alkalosis, uraemia, peripheral vasoconstriction, muscle cramps or oedema. Patients with metabolic alkalosis have shallow respiration, appear irritable and unco-operative.

Table 2.3 Problems associated with prolonged nausea and vomiting

- anorexia
- dehydration
- electrolyte imbalance
- malnutrition
- weakness
- lethargy
- loss of morale

- depression
- Mallory-Weiss tears or damage to the gastrointestinal tract
- fractures
- increased length of hospital stay

For surgical patients

- aspiration of vomitus into the lungs
- wound disruption

For cancer patients

- poor compliance with treatment schedules
- refusal of treatment

Metabolic alkalosis
The body is usually kept at a neutral pH (7.3) by the balance of hydrogen (H^+) and bicarbonate (HCO_3^-) ions. Any situation that removes one of these preferentially will disturb the balance. As gastric juice is very acid, vomiting causes a loss of hydrogen ions, and a rise to metabolic alkalosis as the pH of the body fluids rises towards 8.0. Many physiological processes come into place to restore normal pH. They include increased excretion of bicarbonate, sodium and potassium by the kidney. The clinical symptoms of these events include muscle cramps and fatigue – which are probably due to the loss of sodium and potassium ions – and shallow respiration as alkaline plasma inhibits the respiratory centre.

Violent episodes of vomiting can cause physical injury, such as tears of the gastric mucosa – so called Mallory-Weiss tears (Enck, 1977) or the ruptured oesophagus of Boerhaave's syndrome. Even fractures of the ribs have been reported. These events are very rare and tend to occur more readily in patients who already have some weakness, for example Mallory-Weiss tears are most common in alcoholics.

Mallory-Weiss tears are tears of the mucosa in the lower oesophagus or gastric cardia. They are caused by prolonged and forceful vomiting and can give rise to haematemesis (blood in the vomitus).

Surgical patients can have special problems with nausea and vomiting. There are dangers for a patient who is vomiting while under the influence of anaesthetics. Vomitus can be inhaled and this could prove fatal if the cough reflex is inhibited or depressed. Obviously such patients would not be left unattended but this has been identified as a risk factor after oral surgery where the jaws are wired together (Cookson, 1986). After surgery vomiting can cause pain and disruption of the wound that impairs healing. Delicate surgical work following plastic or ophthalmic surgery is especially vulnerable and bleeding beneath skin flaps (Stein, 1982) or vitreous loss from the eye are serious hazards.

Patients feel undignified and often embarrassed by periods of vomiting; this can give rise to depression and a loss of morale.

These effects can impinge upon an individual's ability to carry out normal daily activities, decreasing quality of life and hindering recovery from illness.

Nausea and vomiting have been reported as the most frequent anaesthetic-related cause for hospitalization of what should be day-case surgery or re-admittance to hospital after discharge. These instances and non-surgical situations where discharge from hospital has been delayed due to nausea and vomiting have important economic consequences.

Probably the most insidious of problems to arise from prolonged nausea and vomiting is that cancer patients can delay coming for treatment beyond the optimum time interval or may refuse treatment altogether.

2.9 The vomiting reflex

The vomiting reflex involves detectors which identify the need to vomit, effectors which cause the vomiting and a co-ordinating centre which will organize the entire process. The need to vomit can be signalled by a toxic substance or by unusual quantities of normal body constituents. For example, high circulating levels of urea can cause vomiting in renal failure. Breakdown products of tissue damage can have the same effect. So, in its simplest form, we can view vomiting as being induced by ingestion of toxins or tissue damage.

The detectors

The body needs detectors to identify the need to vomit. The main detectors of the need to vomit are the gastrointestinal tract, a specialized area of the brain called the chemoreceptor trigger zone (CTZ), the labyrinthine apparatus of the ear and higher brain centres which process the 'emotional' stimuli to vomiting. The CTZ is located in the *area postrema* (AP). This is a bilateral structure located on the floor of the IVth ventricle, at the level of the *obex* (Figure 2.4).

As toxins frequently enter the body by ingestion it is not surprising that there are detectors for toxic chemicals in the stomach and duodenum. These are termed chemoreceptors. They will respond to agents that cause irritation of the mucosa. There are also mechanoreceptors which detect over-distension of the stomach or duodenum and also respond to disordered patterns of gastric motility.

The venous drainage of the gut, at least the stomach and duodenum, is by means of the hepatic portal vein. As blood

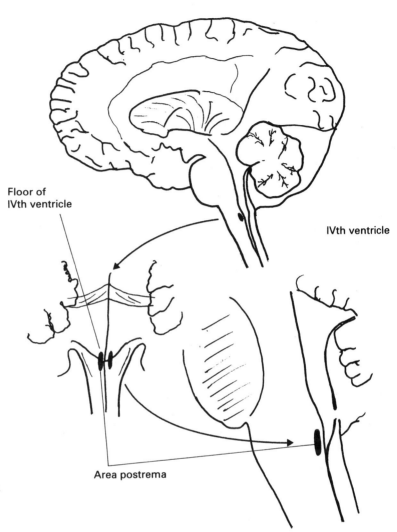

Floor of
IVth ventricle

IVth ventricle

Area postrema

Figure 2.4 The location of the CTZ. The CTZ is on the surface of the brainstem, on the floor of the IVth ventricle.

passes directly to the liver before mixing with the systemic circulation, high concentrations of substances absorbed from the gut will reach the liver. It is possible that hepatic detectors for absorbed chemicals also exist.

If a toxin is absorbed it will enter the systemic circulation after passing through the liver. Detecting these absorbed toxins is the role of the CTZ in the AP.

Although the CTZ is located in the brain it is effectively outside the blood-brain barrier and is, therefore, sensitive to agents circulating in the blood. Since it is on the floor of the IVth ventricle it is in contact with the cerebrospinal fluid (CSF) and will also detect substances in the CSF.

The blood-brain barrier
In order to protect the brain most of its blood vessels have a smooth continuous wall – in histological terms they are said to be non-fenestrated (L. *fenestra* = window, hence no windows). This is shown in Figure 2.5. Many substances, especially large molecules, in the blood cannot, therefore, reach the nerve cells. This relative impermeability of the vessels is referred to as the blood-brain barrier (BBB). Its existence may be especially useful in the case of some drugs that need to act in the periphery but where central actions are undesirable. Several regions exist in the brain where the capillaries are more permeable – they are fenestrated – and thus more substances are able to gain access to the brain. These regions are said to be 'outside' the blood-brain barrier. (This is rather a confusing term – the regions behave as if they were holes in the barrier.) The *area postrema* is one of these regions.

Non-fenestrated capillary

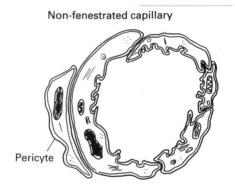

Pericyte

Fenestrated capillary

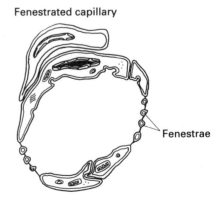

Fenestrae

Figure 2.5 Fenestrated and non-fenestrated capillaries. Non-fenestrated capillaries which are found in the brain are less permeable than fenestrated capillaries.

A toxin entering the body through being ingested has at least three chances of being detected: (i) by the gut; (ii) by the liver, immediately after absorption; or (iii) by the CTZ, on entering the systemic circulation.

If a toxic substance has been injected it will have a fairly rapid action on the CTZ. However, despite its name, this region is probably not the main detector of cytotoxic drugs as these drugs and radiation can also have some very important actions on the gut.

Once receptors (chemoreceptors or mechanoreceptors) in the gastrointestinal tract have been stimulated messages are relayed to the brain by means of the vagus nerve (or more correctly the vagi as the nerve branches into two – a dorsal and ventral portion). There is also an hepatic branch of the vagus which innervates the liver.

> The vagus is a mainly afferent nerve which innervates among other tissues the upper gut and transmits messages to the brain. The vagus, or Xth cranial nerve, is a major nerve of the parasympathetic nervous system.

Messages transmitted by means of the vagus nerve reach the brain at the nucleus of the solitary tract. This is usually abbreviated as NTS (L. *nucleus tractus solitarius*). Some fibres of the vagus also pass to the AP and an adjacent region called the *area subpostrema* (Leslie & Gwyn, 1984). The AP also has direct connections to the NTS. Thus the AP can receive messages through several routes; from the gut, through other branches of the vagus nerve and from the circulation.

So there is quite a complex circuit – an agent could stimulate the gut and cause messages to be relayed directly to the NTS or messages could pass from the gut by means of the CTZ to the NTS, or it could stimulate the CTZ directly. It is possible that a toxin or something like a cytotoxic drug could act at all three sites. Once this has occurred, messages are passed to the next link in the chain – the vomiting centre (Figure 2.6).

The co-ordinator   The co-ordinator of the vomiting process is the vomiting centre (VC). The role of the VC is to orchestrate the whole process of nausea and vomiting. It has to detect the need to vomit and co-ordinate the quite complex sequence of events that cause nausea, retching and culminate in vomiting.

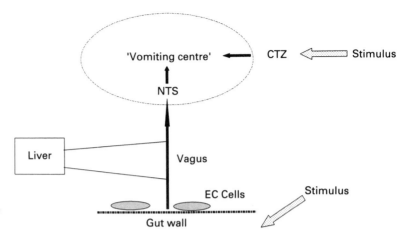

Figure 2.6 Afferent pathways from the gastrointestinal tract to the 'Vomiting Centre'.

The term 'vomiting centre' dates from the early days of physiological studies when a centre was the term used to discuss a discrete brain area controlling a defined process, such as the respiratory centre. The VC was proposed as far back as 1865 by Giannuzzi (Wang & Borison, 1950).

All the processes that occur during vomiting are part of normal bodily activities, e.g. salivation, gastric acid secretion and contraction of the respiratory muscles. What happens during vomiting is that these events occur in a particular pattern and, usually, in a more vigorous fashion than normal.

The VC is then really a functional centre rather than an anatomical centre and, as such, cannot be given precise anatomical boundaries. Current thinking is that the VC is not a 'black box' although the name is a useful shorthand and important aspects of the VC can be identified (Davis *et al.*, 1986). It is located in the brainstem, close to the IVth ventricle in the parvocellular reticular formation and is viewed as a fairly large area of the brainstem encompassing the recipients of the vagal afferent inputs – the NTS and the nuclei controlling the motor events involved in vomiting. These nuclei are the dorsal motor nucleus of the vagus (DMVN), which controls the muscles of the throat and gastrointestinal secretions, the *nucleus ambiguus*, which innervates the muscles of the larynx and pharynx and the ventral respiratory group of neurones which control the respiratory muscles (Figure 2.7).

Thus afferent information will come from the gut via the vagus nerve and the NTS, from the AP, from the vestibular apparatus of the ear and from higher parts of the brain (Figure 2.8). The information will be interpreted and messages sent to many areas of the body.

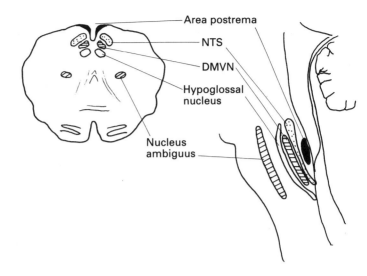

Figure 2.7 Central component of the vomiting reflex. The NTS is the primary recipient of vagal afferent information; the DMVN control the muscles of the throat and the gastrointestinal secretions; the nucleus ambiguus innervates the muscle of the pharynx and larynx; the hypoglossal nucleus controls the movements of the tongue and mouth.

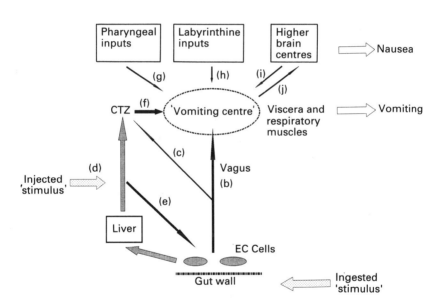

Figure 2.8 Pathways of the vomiting reflex. Ingested toxins may stimulate chemoreceptors or may release 5-HT from the EC cells. This can result in stimulation of the vagus (b). Vagal stimulation directly affects the VC or pathways to the CTZ are stimulated (c). The toxin may be absorbed (a) where it can stimulate hepatic detectors. Injected agents will enter the systemic circulation. Once in the blood agents can affect EC cells (e) or have direct action on the CTZ (d), which is transmitted to the VC (f). Other inputs are from the pharynx (g), labyrinthine apparatus of the ear (h). Higher brain centres can stimulate the VC (i) and information from the VC to higher brain centres is involved in the perception of nausea (j). Once stimulated the VC orchestrates the process of vomiting. (See section 2.12 and 2.13.)

The effectors

The 'output' arm of the vomiting reflex consists of higher brain centres, the motor nerves co-ordinating respiratory muscle movement, the vagal outputs that control gastric acid secretion and sympathetic nerves that cause peripheral vasoconstriction, increased salivation and so on.

The vagal efferent neurones supplying the heart and stomach originate in the DMVN and the *nucleus ambiguus*. The pre-sympathetic neurones which maintain sympathetic tone to the heart and blood vessels are located close by in the ventrolateral brainstem. Dorsal and ventral groups of respiratory neurones are also located here.

2.10 Other pathways involved in vomiting

Although this description has concentrated on gastrointestinal and CTZ pathways, there are other pathways which may stimulate vomiting and may be relevant (Figure 2.9). An important point to remember is that emetic stimuli are additive or cumulative – if one factor is making you feel just a 'bit sick' a second stimulus added to this can actually precipitate vomiting. In the context of patients who are about to undergo treatment, two of the many factors that will predispose them to vomiting are anxiety and pain.

Pharyngeal stimulation can produce vomiting. This is the pathway stimulated when fingers are placed at the back of the throat to induce vomiting – often used when children have swallowed a foreign body.

Higher brain centres – the cortex and limbic system – must

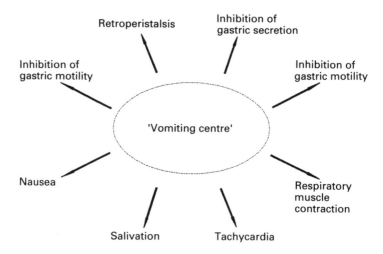

Figure 2.9 Efferent pathways of the vomiting reflex. Once stimulated the VC acts to orchestrate the whole process of vomiting.

have an input to the VC as emotions, sights or thoughts can precipitate vomiting.

Motion can cause vomiting. This results from stimulation of the labyrinthine apparatus of the ear. The vestibulocerebellar pathway (involving the ear and cerebellum) can be the sole cause of vomiting, as in motion sickness, or can be a contributory factor especially where a patient is being moved after some other emetic stimulus; e.g. movement from bed to trolley after surgery or rotation on a table during radiotherapy. As emetic stimuli have an additive effect, movement of a patient may be a contributory factor to patient discomfort.

There is an auricular branch of the vagus nerve which innervates the tympanum of the ear. Also known as Arnold's nerve or the Alderman's nerve, this was used as a readily accessible point to stimulate vomit by the ancient Romans who would retire and stimulate the tympanum with a feather, causing vomiting and making room for continued indulgence!

The vagus nerve also has a cardiac branch which innervates the heart. This may be why heart attacks are often accompanied by nausea and/or vomiting.

Sympathetic activity from some other organs will also stimulate vomiting. In particular distension of the bladder, gallbladder or uterus, either by disease or trauma, can precipitate vomiting. It is often observed that there is a high incidence of postoperative nausea and vomiting associated with gynaecological surgery (see Chapter 3) and procedures requiring uterine dilatation are associated with more emetic sequelae (Dundee *et al.*, 1962).

2.11 Transmitters involved in the emetic reflex

Much research has focused on trying to identify the neurotransmitters involved in the emetic reflex. Unfortunately the problem does not have a simple solution. The AP and NTS, for example, contain a vast number of different transmitters and many peptides. Looking at the pharmacological action of antiemetic drugs, however, has helped in our understanding of which transmitters are important.

Acetylcholine and histamine seem to be important in the vestibular pathway of motion sickness. Thus anticholinergic drugs (e.g. hyoscine) and antihistaminergic drugs (e.g. diphenhydramine; cinnarizine) are useful treatments for travel sickness. However these are poor anti-emetics in other areas such as chemo- or radiotherapy-induced nausea and vomiting and postoperative nausea and vomiting.

Many anti-emetics are dopamine receptor antagonists (see Chapter 4), suggesting a role for dopamine in the emetic pathway. Certainly there are central dopamine D_2 receptors in the CTZ and the NTS and dopamine has direct actions on gastric motility, acting on peripheral dopamine receptors. Thus dopamine receptor antagonists may act on either the central or peripheral dopamine receptors. Some will act at both sites. Others, such as domperidone, cannot cross the blood-brain barrier and so act only at peripheral sites.

Until recently one of the most effective and widely used anti-emetics, especially for radio- and chemotherapy-induced emesis, was metoclopramide. Metoclopramide is primarily a dopamine antagonist. However, it was demonstrated, first in dogs (Gylys *et al.*, 1979) and then in humans (Gralla *et al.*, 1981) that metoclopramide was far more effective against cisplatin-induced vomiting if the dose was substantially increased.

Receptors

Within the body communication between cells is via molecules (neurotransmitters, hormones, growth factors, etc.) which are released from one cell and act on another. A receptor is the recognition site on the receiving cell that recognizes, binds to and is activated by the messenger molecule. When a receptor is activated a biological response occurs. The molecule which binds to a receptor is called a ligand. If the result of binding is the normal biological event associated with that receptor then the ligand is an agonist; if the binding results in inhibition of the normal response it is an antagonist (Figure 2.10).

Sometimes an agent will have different effects in different tissues or when used at different concentrations. Careful examination of the receptors involved has shown that there are subtle differences between them; there are different receptor types. The skill of the pharmacologist comes in designing drugs which only act on one type of receptor, that is drugs which are selective. The more selective a drug, the less likely it is to produce side-effects.

Scientists were also interested in the finding that metoclopramide, a dopamine receptor antagonist, was capable of antagonising 5-hydroxytryptamine (5-HT, serotonin) at the **M** or

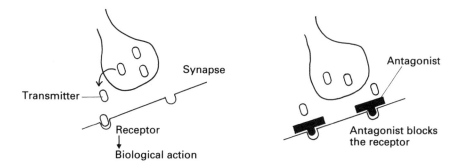

Figure 2.10 Receptors. Specific activation of a receptor by a neurotransmitter results in a biological response. A selective antagonist is capable of blocking the receptors to prevent activation by the normal transmitter.

3 receptor when used in high doses (Fozard & Mobarok-Ali, 1978).

This raised the possibility that it was antagonism of 5-HT rather than antagonism of dopamine that was important in controlling emesis (Miner & Sanger, 1986). Working on this hypothesis several pharmaceutical companies produced drugs designed to act specifically on 5-HT$_3$ receptors.

Research on chemotherapy-induced emesis has relied upon animal models most notably the ferret which responds to cyto-toxic drugs in a similar way to man. By giving anti-emetics, such as metoclopramide, the emesis can be partially controlled (Hawthorn *et al.*, 1988). In this animal model the 5-HT$_3$ receptor antagonists were shown to be capable of totally abolishing the vomiting due to radiation, cisplatin and cyclophosphamide (Costall *et al.*, 1987; Stables *et al.*, 1987; Bermudez *et al.*, 1988).

Cisplatin-induced vomiting
Cisplatin is a cytotoxic drug widely used in chemotherapy regimens. Of all chemotherapeutic drugs it presents perhaps the most challenging clinical problem in terms of nausea and vomiting. Cisplatin will induce emesis in every single patient. The nausea and vomiting are prolonged and severe and delayed emesis lasting several days is not uncommon. The emesis induced by cisplatin is harder to treat than that induced by any other cytotoxic drug. For practical purposes chemotherapy is often divided into cisplatin containing regimens and those without cisplatin which are often termed less emetogenic or moderately emetogenic che-motherapy (see Chapter 3).

The effectiveness of 5-HT$_3$ receptor antagonists, and the location of 5-HT led to the hypothesis that radiotherapy and chemotherapy induce vomiting by causing the release of 5-HT which activates the emetic reflex (see Andrews & Hawthorn, 1988 and Andrews *et al.*, 1989 for summary). This hypothesis has been developed and strengthened by subsequent studies of the 5-HT$_3$ receptor antagonists – see section 2.13. Because of their importance the 5-HT$_3$ receptor antagonists will be considered in detail along with some brief background notes on 5-HT. (See Figure 2.8.)

2.12 5-HT and its receptors

5-HT or serotonin is an amine formed from the amino acid tryptophan (Figure 2.11). Our source of tryptophan is the diet (i.e. it is an essential amino acid).

5-HT is an important neurotransmitter and is also found in platelets where it is involved in blood clotting. The highest concentration of 5-HT, however, is in the enterochromaffin cells of the gut mucosa which contain about 80–90% of the body's 5-HT.

5-HT has a variety of actions on the cardiovascular, respiratory, gastrointestinal and the central nervous systems. It has been called a 'capricious' neurochemical modulator because it can have opposing effects in the same organ. In the cardiovascular system, for example, it acts on nerves or directly on muscle. Thus, depending on the conditions, 5-HT can cause vasoconstriction or vasodilatation. It can also decrease or increase heart rate. 5-HT is involved in the provocation of pain and has been implicated in the induction of sleep and regulation of sleep patterns. 5-HT may affect mood – influencing aggression, anxiety and depression. It is also a prime suspect as a causative agent in migraine and, as has been seen, plays a major role in nausea and vomiting induced by cytotoxic drugs and

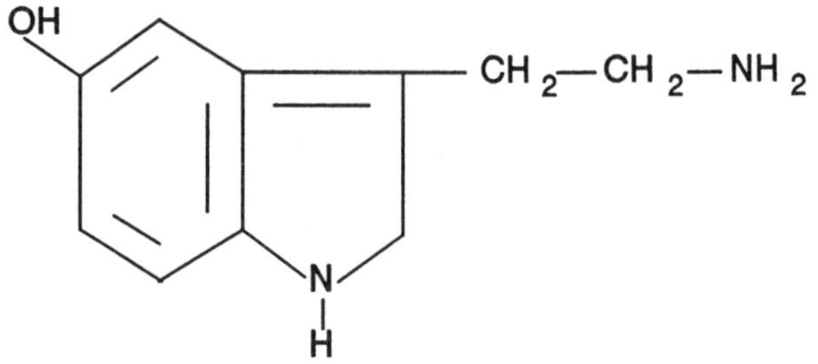

Figure 2.11 5-HT, 5-hydroxytryptamine or serotonin.

radiation. It may also play a role in postoperative nausea and vomiting.

However, it is beyond the scope of this book to discuss in detail the large number of physiological actions of 5-HT. The receptors of interest in nausea and vomiting are the 5-HT$_3$ receptors.

Classification of 5-HT receptors

Classification of 5-HT receptors has historically been complex. Initially two types of receptor were described (Gaddum & Picarelli, 1957), known as 'D' and 'M'. This was followed by the description of two central receptors S$_1$ and S$_2$. The situation grew more confusing as new receptors were described and new agonists and antagonists were synthesized. Each research group was using its own system for naming them. Clearly the confusion over receptors had to be confronted. A meeting of leading 5-HT research workers devised a new system of classification in 1986; at this time three groups of receptors were proposed (1, 2 and 3) and this was universally accepted (Bradley *et al.*, 1986). The number of receptor subtypes has steadily increased since that meeting with some groups being further subdivided as research progressed. The receptor nomenclature was revised in 1993 (Humphrey *et al.*, 1993) when four groups of receptors were accepted. At the time of writing (March 1994) there are seven groups of 5-HT receptors.

It is the 5-HT$_3$ receptor which is involved in vomiting. Some of the earlier anti-emetic studies may refer to the 'M' receptor – this is the same as the '3' receptor.

The 5-HT$_1$ group is subdivided into 1A, 1B, 1D, 1E and 1F. The 5-HT$_2$ group has been subdivided into 2A, 2B, and 2C and there is evidence that even the 5-HT$_3$ receptor may not be a homogeneous population.

2.13 Site of action of 5-HT$_3$ receptor antagonists

It has already been stated that release of 5-HT by chemotherapy or radiotherapy is thought to cause the nausea and vomiting associated with cancer treatment, similarly surgical procedures may release 5-HT giving rise to postoperative symptoms. The most likely explanation is that treatment causes a release of 5-HT probably from the enterochromaffin cells of the gut mucosa. The 5-HT then activates vagal afferent nerve terminals to initiate vomiting. 5-HT$_3$ receptor antagonists block these receptors and prevent information being relayed via the vagus. (See Andrews *et al.*, 1989 for review). It is unlikely that circulating 5-HT has direct actions on the CTZ, since 5-HT is rapidly degraded in plasma and high levels of 5-HT would not reach the CTZ.

Another possible site of action is the 5-HT$_3$ receptors located centrally in the NTS or the *area subpostrema*. If 5-HT is involved in the central processing of information involved in vomiting, blocking 5-HT$_3$ receptors would effectively prevent this and control vomiting. It is quite possible that the 5-HT$_3$ receptor antagonists are acting at both sites.

There are several pieces of important information which must be drawn together to support this hypothesis.

First, 5-HT$_3$ receptors are distributed in the areas of the body involved in vomiting. The highest concentration is on the vagus nerve, especially around the nerve terminals (Ireland & Tyers, 1987). There are in fact 5-HT$_3$ receptors along the length of the vagi and it is thought that these receptors are synthesized in the nodose ganglion, the collection of cell bodies of the vagus, and from there they move along the nerve to the afferent terminals. There is also a high density of 5-HT$_3$ receptors in the brainstem, especially in the NTS and in a region intimately associated with the AP – the *area subpostrema* (Kilpatrick *et al.*, 1988; Pratt *et al.*, 1990). The receptors in the NTS are on pre-synaptic vagal terminals so that blocking these receptors would stop central processing of information that is coming to the CNS from the periphery.

Second, the highest concentration of 5-HT is in the enterochromaffin cells in the mucosa of the gastrointestinal tract. These cells are particularly dense in the duodenum and stomach. Thus if a stimulus is releasing 5-HT the 5-HT will be in exactly the right place to stimulate vagal afferent terminals.

So if we look again at the emetic pathway and consider how 5-HT fits in we can see how emesis is caused by anything which releases 5-HT (Figure 2.12).

Studies have looked at the concentrations of 5-HIAA (5-HIAA is the main metabolite of 5-HT, it is excreted in the urine) in the urine of patients who have received chemotherapy (Cubeddu *et al.*, 1990; Cubeddu, 1993). They showed that the urinary con-

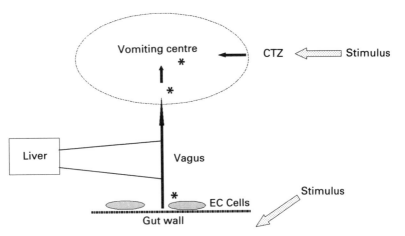

Figure 2.12 Site of action of the 5-HT$_3$ receptor antagonist. The 5-HT$_3$ receptor antagonists may act to block vomiting at vagal afferent terminals, on vagal synapses or other sites in the CNS to prevent processing of emetic stimuli.

centration of 5-HIAA rose after cisplatin or cyclophosphamide treatment compared with healthy controls who received saline. The rise was greatest after cisplatin which is the more emetogenic regimen and less after the less emetogenic drug, cyclophosphamide. This is good circumstantial evidence that 5-HT is involved in the emetic reflex, although it cannot be proved by this experiment that the cytotoxic drugs caused the release of 5-HT. The very act of vomiting will release 5-HT in very large quantities and the amount of emesis experienced by these patients was not recorded. It would be interesting if differences could be seen between patients who vomit and those who do not. The authors themselves also point out that the 5-HIAA release could be due to damage of the mucosal lining which was not related to the nausea and vomiting.

This could help to explain why so many diverse drugs and stimuli have the same common end point – vomiting. This explanation may be an oversimplification. It is likely that vomiting is a complex process involving more than one single transmitter. Maybe 5-HT is acting in concert with another factor. The fact that 5-HT$_3$ receptor antagonists are so good at controlling emesis shows that 5-HT has a pivotal role.

These drugs have proved so successful in controlling certain types of vomiting that they have revolutionized certain areas of nursing, most notable the ability to control the side effect of vomiting in cancer patients. Better anti-emetic control has also allowed higher doses of cytotoxic drugs to be given.

A curious paradox exists. Patients who suffer from carcinoid syndrome possess a tumour that secretes excessive amounts of 5-HT but they do not display unusual amounts of nausea and vomiting. It may be that where the 5-HT is released is just as important as how much is produced. That is large amounts of 5-HT released from enterochromaffin cells will be in the mucosa, close to vagal afferent endings. Circulating 5-HT, on the other hand, is on the serosal side of the gut wall.

Furthermore, the 5-HT₃ receptor antagonists provide both effective therapeutic agents and useful experimental tools allowing us to define even more clearly what is happening in the emetic pathway.

The following chapter will consider how nausea and vomiting is caused by a variety of different stimuli.

Summary of Chapter 2

- The physiology of nausea and vomiting is not completely understood. In biological terms vomiting serves to protect an organism from ingesting poisons but it is clearly more complex than this. Vomiting can have psychological causes as well as physiological causes.
- Nausea usually precedes vomiting. It is an unpleasant subjective sensation, associated with changes in the gut.
- Retching is breathing in against a closed glottis.
- Vomiting is the forceful expulsion of the gastric contents.
- The detectors of the need to vomit in response to chemotherapy and radiotherapy are the gut and the chemoreceptor trigger zone (CTZ).
- Vomiting is co-ordinated by an area of the brainstem called the 'vomiting centre' (VC). It is effected by the respiratory muscles along with changes in the gut.
- Chemo- and radiotherapy probably cause vomiting by releasing a large amount of 5-HT from the enterochromaffin cells in the gastrointestinal mucosa. This then acts on nearby vagal afferent terminals.
- Vomiting after surgery is probably due in part to release of 5-HT.

- 5-HT$_3$ receptor antagonists may act on vagal afferent terminals or in areas such as the CTZ or nucleus of the solitary tract (NTS) to prevent central processing of information received from other regions of the body.
- Vomiting has a variety of consequences, both physiological and psychological; for some patient groups effects on patient morale may be as important as physiological effects.

SELF ASSESSMENT QUESTIONS

1. The following changes are associated
   with nausea:

   TRUE   FALSE

   (a) increased gastric acid secretion
   (b) increased salivation
   (c) increased gut motility
   (d) increase of sympathetic nervous
       activity

2. Retching involves:

   (a) the respiratory muscles
   (b) decreased abdominal pressure
   (c) movement of gut contents from
       duodenum to stomach
   (d) a closed glottis

3. The main detectors involved in
   chemotherapy-induced vomiting are:

   (a) the gut
   (b) the chemoreceptor trigger zone (CTZ)
   (c) the 'vomiting centre'
   (d) all three

4. The vagus innervates:

   (a) the heart
   (b) the lungs
   (c) the liver
   (d) the kidneys
   (e) the upper gastrointestinal tract

5. The area postrema (AP) contains:

   (a) The CTZ
   (b) the 'vomiting centre'
   (c) both the CTZ and the 'vomiting centre'

6. Which of the following are true?
   (mark one or more boxes with a tick):   TRUE   FALSE

   (a) the CTZ is inside the blood-brain
       barrier (BBB)
   (b) gastric stasis is associated with nausea
   (c) the 'vomiting centre' is a co-ordinating
       centre
   (d) the limbic system can stimulate the
       'vomiting centre'
   (e) there is a low incidence of vomiting
       after gynaecological surgery

7. Motion sickness is best controlled by:

   (a) anti-cholinergic drugs
   (b) anti-dopaminergic drugs
   (c) anti-histaminergic drugs
   (d) anti-serotoninergic drugs

8. 5-HT_3 receptors have been found:

   (a) in the area subpostrema
   (b) in the gut
   (c) in the CTZ
   (d) in the NTS

9. Receptor occupancy gives rise to a
   biological response when:

   (a) it is occupied by an agonist
   (b) it is occupied by an antagonist
   (c) it is occupied by the natural ligand

CHAPTER 3: AETIOLOGY OF NAUSEA AND VOMITING

The previous chapter has described what we know about how the emetic reflex is organized.

Whatever the stimulus the subsequent events of retching and vomiting are the same. The onset and severity of nausea, however, are less clearly definable and can vary greatly with the nature of the stimulus. This chapter seeks to place the physiology in a clinical context so that the underlying causes of nausea and vomiting in a variety of different circumstances can be understood.

There is no doubt that different individuals have a different susceptibility to vomiting. As one nurse summed up: 'some people are just "sickie" people'. This may be due to the patient's own psychological predisposition and/or there may be individual variations in the threshold of the vomiting reflex. As people vary in their ability to tolerate pain or suffer discomfort so the level of stimulus which precipitates vomiting will vary. These variations cannot always be measured but several factors have been identified. Another aspect covered in this chapter is how patient demography influences nausea and vomiting; these characteristics are particularly important in patient responses to radio- and chemotherapy and to postoperative nausea and vomiting.

3.1 Vomiting in babies

It is not unusual for babies to regurgitate some milk after a feed. Often the milk is brought up along with 'wind' or the air that has been swallowed during feeding. Such vomiting, termed possetting, is normal and should not give cause for concern.

Sometimes babies vomit a large proportion of their feed. This can mean that they do not obtain adequate nutrition, may fail to gain weight and will become irritable and cry a great deal. This is a cause for concern and further investigations are necessary.

As with adults, babies can vomit because of an infection. Infections may be very serious, such as meningitis, or due to more common childhood illnesses such as chicken pox or measles.

Babies can also suffer from eating contaminated food in a similar way to adults or the baby may be allergic to, or intolerant of, a component of its food. Allergies may be accompanied by other signs such as rashes. For bottle-fed babies a change of formula may be all that is necessary. Allergy to cow's milk is not uncommon and soya milk based formula should be tried. For breastfed babies the mother may be eating some food that is passing into her milk. Again the culprit may be cow's milk and the mother may find that eliminating milk from her own diet will help the baby.

It is essential that the baby is given plenty of fluids and that the baby's diet is investigated as soon as possible. An anxious mother, or one who is in poor health, may have difficulty breastfeeding and may need some help with the technique or encouragement to supplement her own milk with baby formula. The help of an experienced midwife or trained breastfeeding counsellor may be useful.

In some cases a baby may develop projectile vomiting when three to four weeks old. The feed may be ejected a distance of several feet. This is due to a thickening of the pyloric muscle which occurs for unknown reasons after birth (Figure 3.1). The pylorus becomes narrowed and forceful vomiting is the result. The condition, known as pyloric stenosis, can be confirmed by abdominal examination when the thickened pylorus can be palpated. A barium meal may be required to confirm the diagnosis. The usual treatment in babies is by surgery when an incision is made along the thickened muscle.

Any baby who is vomiting frequently must be seen by a doctor.

3.2 Motion sickness

There are numerous circumstances in which motion sickness can occur; sea sickness, car sickness, swing sickness, space sickness, cinerama sickness and, most recently, people using virtual reality headsets report feeling 'travel sick'. What is noticeable is that while most forms are due to actual physical motion there are circumstances where motion sickness can occur even though the subject is stationary. If someone stands in a room and the scenery is moved around them they may well feel motion sickness.

These observations have helped to identify the important component of motion sickness and the development of the

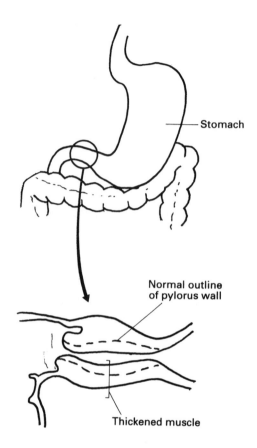

Stomach

Normal outline
of pylorus wall

Thickened muscle

Figure 3.1 Pyloric
stenosis. The muscle wall
at the pyloric sphincter is
abnormally thickened.

'sensory conflict theory'. This theory was proposed as long ago
as 1881 by Irwin and has been consolidated and developed ever
since, notably by Reason (1970). When the body is in motion the
outside world is sensed through the visual system and at the
same time the vestibular system responds sensing angular
changes through the semi-circular canals and acceleration
through the otoliths. The sensory conflict theory proposes that
motion sickness occurs when the information coming from
these structures does not agree. For example, if the eyes sense
movement but the ears are not receiving the same input there
will be conflict. Travelling in cars or especially in boats produces movement that the ears do not interpret in the same way
as do the eyes. Travel sickness in a boat is usually worse when
the subject is below decks where the environment is static
relative to the subject. Going above deck so that the person can
see the movement of the horizon often helps relieve nausea and
vomiting. This is a simplified explanation and a more detailed
discussion of the topic is given by Stott (1986).

In the clinical situation motion can contribute to the sickness experience by any patients who are being moved. Being wheeled along while lying down is a particularly potent stimulus and can precipitate feelings of nausea. Radiotherapy patients can be distressed by being rotated in the radiotherapy apparatus. Any patient travelling home after treatment can be susceptible to travel sickness especially if their treatment has already made them feel nauseous, for example cancer patients having received chemotherapy.

3.3 Vomiting due to disease

Gastrointestinal disease

Diseases of the gastrointestinal tract cause nausea and/or vomiting by stimulating the vagal afferent pathway. The stimuli can be broadly divided into those affecting the chemoreceptor or those affecting the mechanoreceptors. However, many stimuli will affect both sorts of receptors. Chemoreceptors can be irritated by components of the diet or by inflammation of the gastrointestinal mucosa.

Excess alcohol or spicy foods rich in capsaicin (the 'hot' component of chillies) can inflame the mucosa as can drugs such as aspirin. Inflammation may be due to infection such as gastroenteritis or the more serious conditions of peptic or duodenal ulcer or gastric carcinoma. Appendicitis can cause nausea and vomiting.

Obstruction will cause over-distension of the stomach and/or small intestine and thus evoke vomiting. The causes of obstruction may be a tumour; carcinoma of the pancreas frequently presents with nausea and vomiting as a major symptom. Ovarian tumours may press on the neighbouring bowel and cause an obstruction.

Pyloric stenosis presents with symptoms similar to those seen in young babies, that is forceful projectile vomiting of large quantities of vomitus. Often items of food ingested several hours before can be identified in the vomitus of patients with obstructions.

Mechanoreceptors will also be stimulated by disordered motility patterns such as the stasis associated with diabetes (diabetic gastroparesis). Coeliac disease can cause disordered motility.

Constipation and a low-level of motility in the bowel can cause nausea and (less commonly) vomiting.

Other diseases and drugs

Raised intracranial pressure (ICP) can cause nausea and vomiting and in such cases the underlying pathology may be serious. Intracranial pressure can be elevated by infections such as meningitis or encephalitis, by tumours or trauma. A cerebrovascular accident or subarachnoid haemorrhage can cause increased intracranial pressure.

Reye's syndrome, which usually occurs in children under 15 years old, is accompanied by uncontrollable vomiting. This rare syndrome characteristically develops after an upper respiratory tract infection, influenza or chicken pox. It is often associated with taking aspirin to reduce the fever of these illnesses (for this reason paracetamol is currently preferred to aspirin under such circumstances). The features of Reye's syndrome are cerebral oedema and liver damage both of which will cause nausea and vomiting.

Diseases causing unnaturally elevated levels of normal body constituents can also cause nausea and vomiting. The commonest examples are uraemia (elevated levels of blood urea), due to poor renal function, or hypercalcaemia (elevated blood calcium). The latter is often associated with cancers which metastasise to bone. Hypercalcaemia is often accompanied by a dry mouth, drowsiness and confusion and a degree of dehydration.

Diseases of the ear, such as tinnitus or Ménière's disease, can stimulate the labyrinthine pathway and cause nausea and vomiting. Migraine sufferers also experience nausea and vomiting.

Infections can cause nausea and vomiting. Urinary tract infections in particular cause nausea and vomiting especially in children or the terminally ill.

Patients with AIDS experience nausea and vomiting. As they are usually undergoing complex treatment regimens it is difficult to establish whether the vomiting is due to the drugs they are receiving or the underlying pathology of their disease. Drugs such as zidovudine, ganciclovir, acyclovir and co-trimoxazole, which are given to AIDS patients all cause nausea and vomiting.

Other drugs which commonly cause nausea and vomiting are antibiotics, the newer types of antidepressants which act by inhibiting the reuptake of serotonin (selective serotonin reuptake inhibitors or SSRIs), narcotic analgesics and anti-Parkinsonian drugs.

Some of these drugs have obvious actions – SSRIs raise serotonin levels and anti-Parkinsonian drugs elevate central dopamine levels. However the actions of antibiotics and anti-viral drugs are not so obvious. There is a parallel with the action of some of the cytotoxic drugs used in cancer chemotherapy: procarbazine, mustine, cyclophosphamide, chlorambucil, busulphan, cisplatin and some antibiotics all prevent normal DNA transcription. Although we cannot identify how this interruption of cell replication causes emesis there may well be a similar underlying mechanism (see below).

Vomiting in the terminally ill

About one-third of the patients who are referred for hospice care due to terminal cancer will be suffering from nausea and vomiting (Finlay, 1991). The causes of nausea and vomiting in these patients are not different physiologically from those in other patients but some conditions are more prevalent in the terminally ill. These patients are also likely to be suffering from more than one condition which will stimulate the emetic reflex. This exacerbates their symptoms and can make the nausea and vomiting more difficult to control especially if it not realized that there may be more than one underlying cause of the problem.

Gastrointestinal obstruction is a common cause of nausea and vomiting in terminal patients and may be due to a primary tumour of the gastrointestinal tract or large tumour bulk in the abdomen (e.g. ovary) pressing on the gut.

Patients with a grossly enlarged liver, due to metastases, usually have severe nausea with little vomiting. If the liver causes obstruction of the gastric outlet, delays gastric emptying or squashes the stomach huge volumes of undigested food may be vomited. Ascites produces similar symptoms.

Deranged metabolism of advanced cancers or non-specific tissue damage which is still occurring subsequent to recent aggressive radiotherapy or chemotherapy can give rise to unusually elevated levels of intracellular constituents or metabolic products which are detected as 'foreign' by the body and cause nausea and vomiting.

Bony metastases result in elevated levels of blood calcium and hypercalcaemia is a well-known stimulus of nausea and vomiting.

Terminally ill patients are likely to be receiving analgesics on a regular basis. Morphine has a direct emetogenic action and also causes gastric stasis and constipation; both contribute to feelings of nausea.

Raised ICP due to recent radiotherapy of the head and neck or direct pressure from brainstem metastases can stimulate the CTZ.

Many patients with advanced cancer have increased sensitivity to odours (hyperosmia). The mechanism is unknown but strong odours may produce feelings of nausea more readily in these patients.

These factors are summarized in Table 3.1.

Understanding the cause of the nausea and vomiting is essential for choosing the correct anti-emetics. A useful flow diagram to assist this process is given by Regnard and Comiskey (1992).

Table 3.1 Factors causing nausea and vomiting in the terminally ill

---

- gastrointestinal obstruction – due to tumours of the gastrointestinal tract or adjacent tumours
- hepatic metastases
- ascites
- squashed stomach syndrome
- raised intracranial pressure
- drugs e.g. morphine
- hypercalcaemia
- elevated levels of intracellular constituents or metabolites in blood

---

3.4 Vomiting due to cancer treatments: radiotherapy and/or chemotherapy

The nausea and vomiting induced by cancer therapy is prolonged and can be very debilitating. In patients already weakened and perhaps depressed by their disease it is important to avoid further emotional and physical stress. It has been shown to be a major concern for cancer patients (Coates *et al.*, 1983) and can affect their quality of life. For cancer nurses, caring for patients with severe nausea and vomiting can be a source of emotional distress and impinge greatly on nursing time.

Unfortunately the fact that most cancer treatments cause vomiting is common knowledge; patients arrive expecting that they are going to be sick. This only creates anxiety which compounds the problem and presents even more of a challenge for the nurse. If a patient is experiencing pain, such as the deep and intractable pain of bony metastases, this too will become a contributory factor. It is important that nurses, therefore, consider the entire range of possible contributory factors.

These topics have been covered to some extent in Chapter 2 since it is not possible to discuss the physiology of nausea and vomiting without a discussion of how some of the emetic stimuli exert their effects.

Radiotherapy

Radiotherapy generally produces vomiting that is less severe than that associated with aggressive chemotherapy. The number of episodes, however, may be considerably greater than with chemotherapy as a course of radiation treatment can involve 30 or 40 treatments over six to eight weeks. Most radiotherapy techniques deliberately use fractionated doses of 2–3 Gray (Gy), spread over several weeks rather than one large dose as this has been shown to decrease the problems of nausea and vomiting (Priestman, 1988).

A recent development in radiotherapy is CHART (Continuous Hyperfractionated Accelerated Radiotherapy Treatment) where therapy is given at eight-hourly intervals on 12 consecutive days. CHART has been shown to produce a better tumour response than conventional radiotherapy but such intense treatment is likely to increase the amount of nausea and vomiting. If such regimens become widely used the need for an effective anti-emetic in radiotherapy units may well increase.

Several factors influence the susceptibility of a radiotherapy patient to nausea and vomiting (Priestman, 1988). These are considered in the next section.

Main factors predisposing to nausea and vomiting with radiotherapy

Table 3.2 Factors predisposing to nausea and vomiting with radiotherapy

- Site of irradiation
- Field size
- Dose per fraction
- Age
- Anxiety

Site

Irradiation of the upper abdomen (whether irradiated from the front or back) and pelvic region cause most nausea and vomiting. Head and neck irradiation is also quite a potent stimulus whereas therapy to the limbs does not produce much emesis.

Field size

The greater the volume of tissue irradiated the greater the risk of nausea and vomiting. Thus TBI (total body irradiation) is far more emetogenic than focused irradiation of a small region of the body.

Dose per fraction The higher the dose of radiation, the greater the amount of vomiting. This is taken into account when a course of fractionated radiotherapy is designed. Radiotherapy is generally not emetic when the dose is kept below 2–3 Gy.

Age Children appear to experience less sickness than adults.

Anxiety More anxious and apprehensive patients develop more nausea and vomiting.

Chemotherapy As discussed in chapter 2 it is not possible to say unequivocally how cytotoxic drugs act to cause nausea and vomiting. Because the chemoreceptor trigger zone is so named there is the temptation to assume that it is the major detector of drugs used in chemotherapy and hence the site of action whereby these drugs induce nausea and vomiting. However, this is too simple an interpretation and there is a body of evidence which suggests that the gastrointestinal tract is an important site of action of cytotoxic drugs.

Only a brief summary will be given here and the reader is referred to the review by Andrews & Davis (1993) for a detailed evaluation of the subject.

Vomiting can be induced by introducing cisplatin directly into the IVth ventricle, so an involvement of the CTZ cannot be excluded; but drugs which are known to act on the AP have an almost instantaneous effect, e.g. apomorphine given intravenously will cause vomiting within a minute. Cytotoxic drugs on the other hand show a delay or latency to induce emesis often up to several hours. Emesis begins long after drug plasma levels of some cytotoxics have peaked and, in the case of cisplatin, when blood levels have fallen to <10% of initial levels (Carl *et al.*, 1989). However, it may be tissue rather than blood levels of the drugs that are important; considering only circulating drug levels may be misleading.

Sectioning the abdominal vagi can abolish the emetic response to cisplatinum and there is evidence that the abdominal nerves are crucial in the emetic reflex (see Andrews *et al.*, 1990b). Some experiments have concluded that ablation of the AP can abolish the vomiting induced by cisplatinum but as the abdominal vagus also projects to the AP, ablation of this structure could be removing inputs from the periphery to the CNS (see Andrews & Davis, 1993).

There is a protein in neural tissue which is induced in response to neural activity. Using this protein as a marker it has been shown that cisplatinum increases activity of both the NTS and in the AP. However administration of the 5-HT$_3$ receptor antagonist granisetron, at a dose that completely inhibits cisplatin-induced vomiting, significantly reduced activity only in the NTS (Reynolds *et al.*, 1991), demonstrating that activation of the vagal-NTS pathway is important for cisplatin-induced vomiting.

Furthermore, using sensitive binding techniques it has been shown that the 5-HT$_3$ receptors in the NTS are on the terminals of the vagus nerve (Leslie *et al.*, 1990). Thus giving a 5-HT$_3$ receptor antagonist can block the central processing of information coming to the CNS from the abdomen.

Main factors predisposing to nausea and vomiting with chemotherapy

For chemotherapy-induced nausea and vomiting there is considerable variation between the emetic potential of different cytotoxic drugs and between the responses of individual patients to the same drug during different courses of therapy. More aggressive therapy is probably employed where cure is possible but even patients receiving palliative care will still be given emetogenic drugs. The underlying disease may also be causing some degree of sickness. The final outcome is, therefore, a complex computation between the type of cytotoxic drug used, the dosage, how it is administered and the individual patient's response.

The most important determining factor in relation to the amount of sickness experienced by chemotherapy patients is the drugs used. Cisplatin is notorious for the amount of nausea and vomiting it causes, to the extent that some healthcare professionals are likely to regard treatments in two groups: with cisplatin or without. But this division is too crude. Consideration of the effects of non-cisplatin chemotherapy shows that the wide range of cytotoxic drugs can be grouped according to emetic potential. Table 3.3 shows such divisions as reported by Lindley *et al.* (1989).

It must be noted that emetic potential is not determined just by the nature of the drug – the dose used and route of administration will also influence how it affects the patient. For example, cyclophosphamide given orally is in group I whereas a dose of over 1 gm iv is in group V. Most chemotherapy consists

Table 3.3 Emetic potential of cytotoxic drugs (Modified from Lindley, Bernard and Fields, 1989).

Class I Low (<10%)	Class II Moderately Low (10–30%)	Class III Moderate (30–60%)	Class IV Moderately High (60–90%)	Class V High (>90%)
vincristine	methotrexate	cyclopho-	cisplatin	cisplatin
busulfan	<100 mg	sphamide	<75 mg/m²	⩾ 75 mg/m²
chlorambucil	fluorouracil	<1 g	dacarbazine	dacarbazine
thioguanine	⩽ 1000 mg	methotrexate	⩽ 500 mg	⩾ 500 mg
(oral)	doxorubicin	<250 ⩾ 100	cyclophosphamide	cyclophos
cyclophosphamide	cytarabine	doxorubicin	cytarabine	>1 g
(oral)	<20 mg	<75 ⩾ 20	250 mg–1 g	cytarabine
thiotepa	bleomycin	fluorouracil	carmustine	>1 g
	etoposide	⩾ 1000 mg	<200 mg	carmustine
	melphalan	vinblastine	lomustine	⩾ 200 mg
		teniposide	<60 mg	streptozotocin
		azacitidine	doxorubicin	pentostatin
		asparaginase	⩾ 75 mg	mechlorethamine
		cytosine		lomustine ⩾ 60 mg
		methotrexate		
		⩾ 250 mg		
		mitomycin		
		procarbazine		
		anthracyclines		

of a combination of drugs and it is usually the drug with the highest emetic potential which will determine the emetogenicity of the treatment as a whole. These groupings are based on empirical observation and are not the results of comparative trials. Individual nurses may find, therefore, that their own experience of chemotherapy does not quite fit this table. For example, some nurses would place anthracycline in the moderately high rating.

What governs the emetic potential of a cytotoxic drug is not known. It is difficult to find similarities between drugs of similar emetic potential. They cannot be related chemically and do not display the same mechanism of action in attacking cancer cells. Maybe there is an underlying similarity in action in that all of these drugs ultimately arrest cell division. An important point is that even the same dose of drug, given under similar circumstances, will have different emetic potential in different patients – this is where the influence of patient risk factors is seen. The patient risk factors are summarized in Table 3.4.

Table 3.4   Factors predisposing to nausea and vomiting with chemotherapy

- gender
- age
- alcohol intake
- motion sickness
- previous pregnancy
  sickness
- course of treatment
- poor anti-emetic control in
  the past
- anxiety
- treatment setting

Gender and age

Women are more prone to vomiting than men (Zook and Yasko, 1983; Roila *et al.*, 1988) and younger patients are more susceptible (Roila *et al.*, 1988; 1989). Young patients are also more susceptible to the side effects of certain anti-emetics. When drugs that act on the dopamine receptor (e.g. prochlorperazine, metoclopramide) are given they can induce a variety of unwanted extrapyramidal or acute dystonic reactions. These reactions are more pronounced in children and young adults (Kris *et al.*, 1983; Bateman *et al*, 1989). This must be borne in mind when assessing the anti-emetic prescription for these groups of patients.

Alcohol intake

A history of high alcohol intake will reduce the likelihood of a patient suffering from nausea and vomiting after chemotherapy. It is a history of high alcohol intake and not current drinking levels that are important (D'Aquisto *et al.*, 1986). What changes have occurred in the heavy drinker are not known but these are presumably subtle irreversible changes leading to a blunted response. One study (which perhaps did not appreciate this latter point) investigated using intravenous ethanol as an anti-emetic. In this study of patients receiving cisplatin ethanol proved inferior to metoclopramide as an anti-emetic (Spiess *et al.*, 1987).

Motion sickness

Patients with a history of motion sickness have been reported to experience more nausea and vomiting (Morrow, 1985) although the effect was modest.

Previous pregnancy sickness

Women who had suffered sickness during past pregnancies were evaluated for their response to chemotherapy for breast cancer. It was found that those with a higher grade of pregnancy sickness had more chemotherapy-induced vomiting (Martin & Diaz-Rubio, 1990).

Cycle of treatment   The cycle of treatment will influence the degree of nausea and vomiting. The number of patients completely free of nausea and vomiting decreases as the treatment continues (Roila *et al.*, 1989) and major control of emesis is three times more likely in patients on their first course of chemotherapy than in those who have received chemotherapy before (Gralla *et al.*, 1981). It is clearly important to pay particular attention to patients receiving chemotherapy for the first time as the pattern can be set for future courses of treatment. Inadequate anti-emetic control at this stage can produce distress and anxiety that is carried on to the next stage of treatment. It can create expectations of unpleasant treatment sessions that become self-fulfilling and may even predispose the patient to developing anticipatory symptoms (see below).

Indeed there are several identifiable psychological factors which will increase the amount of nausea and vomiting a patient can experience. Any actor or performer who has felt nauseous, or even vomited, before a performance will testify to the fact that psychological input alone can initiate the vomiting reflex.

Anxiety   Anxiety, stress and the patient's own expectations of post-treatment nausea and vomiting are the most widely investigated psychological factors (Jacobsen *et al.*, 1988; Carey & Burish, 1988). Anxiety is generally accepted to exacerbate post-treatment symptoms (Andrykowski & Gregg, 1992). Studies have shown that state anxiety is significantly related to both severity and incidence of nausea (Jacobsen *et al.*, 1988; Andry-kowski & Gregg, 1992). However, Rhodes *et al.*, (1986) showed that state anxiety assessed the morning following chemotherapy was unrelated to post-treatment vomiting but related to post-treatment nausea. Zook and Yasko (1983) also could not relate state anxiety to post-treatment nausea and vomiting. This discrepancy in results may be due to the time at which anxiety was assessed. The Rhodes study assessed patients the following morning and the Zook study assessed patients sometime during the 24 hours before treatment – if anxiety is having a direct effect on gastrointestinal function then it may be important to measure anxiety at the same time as the patient receives their infusion; an assessment made at a different time may not identify all patients who were feeling anxious during the infusion. The latter authors also conclude themselves that their sample was small and the subjects had very low levels of anxiety.

Treatment setting Anti-emetic control has been demonstrated to be less efficient in outpatient settings than in hospitals (Roila *et al.*, 1989). The reasons for this are not clear but it is possible that there is more time available for the assessment of risk factors in an inpatient setting than in a clinic where the treatment nurse may not have a lot of opportunity to investigate the risk factors for a particular patient before treatment begins.

Timing of emesis There is scant information about the time of onset (or latency) of vomiting and even less on nausea. In some ways this is not surprising as few patients will be given treatment without concomitant anti-emetics and anti-emetic medication will modify the latency considerably.

The timing of radiotherapy-induced emesis is poorly documented. One study reports that patients receiving radiation to pelvic and posterior spinal fields vomited 1–6 hours later (30% within three hours) (Welch, 1980).

The latency of chemotherapy varies considerably with different drugs. Agents such as carmustine or lomustine induce vomiting 30 minutes to two hours after their administration. With cisplatin the problem may occur four to eight hours after treatment. Cyclophosphamide induced vomiting does not usually occur until 9–18 hours after the start of chemotherapy.

The onset and duration of vomiting for the commonly used drugs have been summarized by Triozzi and Laszlo (1987) and is reproduced in Table 3.5. Clinical experience would suggest that the latency for cisplatin is much longer than one hour and

Table 3.5 Onset and duration of emesis produced by common cytotoxic drugs

Cisplatin	(1–72 h)
Dacarbazine	(1–12 h)
Mustine	(30 min–36 h)
Doxorubicin	(2–48 h)
Daunorubicin	(2–48 h)
Cyclophosphamide	(8–24 h)
Nitrosoureas	(2–24 h)
Procarbazine	(8–24 h)
Mitomycin C	(1–72 h)
Dactinomycin	(12–24 h; occasionally immediate)

(Adapted from: Triozzi and Laszlo, 1987)

the duration of vomiting with many of these agents is longer than 72 hours. Cancer nurses will find many variations from these times in their own experience, depending on a variety of factors, but this table serves as a useful guide.

In particular, the duration of nausea and emesis varies in different patients. Some individuals will have periods of nausea and vomiting over several days. This delayed nausea and emesis is considered in more detail below.

As most chemotherapy regimens involve a combination or cocktail of cytotoxic drugs the picture may be even more complex. However, it is probably fair to assume that some degree of nausea and vomiting will occur in the majority of patients. Situations will vary but a generalized picture of post-chemotherapy vomiting may be summarized as follows.

Nausea and vomiting will usually begin within four hours of administration of chemotherapy. They reach a peak within the first 4–10 hours and begin to subside after 12–24 hours although some effects can continue for days or weeks. This is particularly true for nausea.

Repeated administration of chemotherapy over consecutive days shows a different pattern. Nausea and vomiting tend to peak on the first day and continue, slightly abated, on the second day. As therapy continues the side effects subside and the patient may even feel quite well and hungry by day 4 or 5.

However, if repeat courses of chemotherapy are given, with several non-treatment days intervening, the pattern of nausea and vomiting is similar to – or even more severe – than that experienced during the first cycle of chemotherapy. Some patterns of vomiting with or without anti-emetic drugs are shown in Figure 3.2.

Acute and delayed nausea and vomiting

The nausea and vomiting which occurs during the first 24 hours following chemotherapy is termed acute nausea and vomiting or emesis. That which occurs during the subsequent days is termed delayed nausea and vomiting or emesis. (While not strictly correct, these terms usually appear in the literature abbreviated to acute emesis and delayed emesis.) This distinction is one of convenience and is usually related to how treatment is documented – the day of treatment and subsequent days are listed as day 1, 2 or 3 after treatment.

What is usually seen is a pattern of decreasing incidence and severity of nausea and vomiting over time, so that delayed emesis is not as severe as acute emesis. Delayed symptoms are most

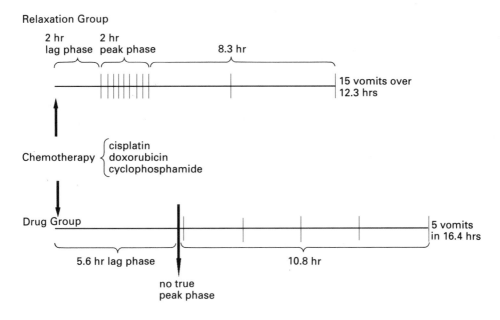

Figure 3.2 Patterns of vomiting (data from Scott *et al.*, 1986).

common after cisplatin but also occur with ifosfamide and cyclo-phosphamide-containing therapy. Investigations of delayed emesis have not always been as thorough as those relating to acute emesis therefore it is difficult to say with certainty how large a problem delayed emesis presents. It has been reported that between 20% and 93% of patients have nausea and/or vomiting during the days following treatment. Even this may not be a true picture as out-patients will not always give accurate reports of their experiences; sometimes they forget, or nobody actually asks about such symptoms. Delayed symptoms can have a great impact on the patient's quality of life. Someone who is feeling nauseous for days will find keeping a job or running a home extremely difficult. Constant nausea and/or vomiting will contribute to the development of anticipatory nausea and vomiting and may also result in poor compliance with treatment schedules.

Even when patients do not have acute nausea and vomiting they may still suffer from delayed symptoms. It was found in one study (Kris *et al.*, 1985a) that the majority of patients who had enjoyed complete control of nausea and emesis during the 24 hours after chemotherapy with cisplatin later went on to develop nausea and emesis during the subsequent 2–4 days. The peak period for delayed nausea and emesis in this group was 48–72 hours (Figure 3.3).

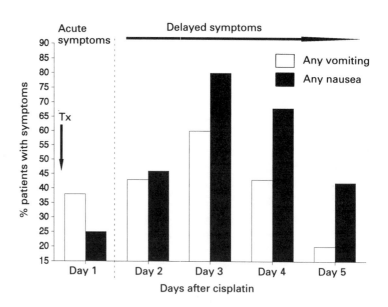

Figure 3.3 The pattern of delayed vomiting following cisplatin. Delayed symptoms, especially nausea may be more severe on days 2 and 3 than on the day of treatment. Patients received metoclopramide, dexamethasone and lorazepam or diphenhydramine on day 1. (Modified from Kris *et al.*, 1985a).

Since delayed emesis can last for several days it is important that anti-emetic therapy is not curtailed too soon. It has been noted that while the 5-HT$_3$ receptor antagonists provide a much better control of acute emesis that is unprecedented with any other anti-emetics this superiority is not always maintained over the days following highly emetogenic chemotherapy, when the efficacy of the 5-HT$_3$ receptor antagonists is similar to that seen with other anti-emetics (Jones *et al.*, 1991; Venner, 1990). This has lead to speculation that other mechanisms besides 5-HT release may be operating during the delayed phase. Andrews and Davis (1993) have suggested that the initial effects of cyto-toxic drugs in releasing 5-HT may be followed by a prolonged phase of tissue damage which releases other emetogenic sub-stances besides 5-HT. This damage could possibly be slowed by the use of steroids, which are known to have actions on stabi-lizing cell membranes. This would divide emesis into a phase which is best controlled by 5-HT$_3$ receptor antagonists and a steroid sensitive phase where the presence of steroids have important effects (Figure 3.4).

It must be remembered that clinical studies have used a fairly arbitrary demarcation between acute and delayed symptoms at 24 hours. We should not think of one mechanism being responsible for emesis during the first 24 hours after che-motherapy which switches off and then another mechanism takes over, which is responsible for delayed emesis. Perhaps we should think of the emetic response being due to a number of

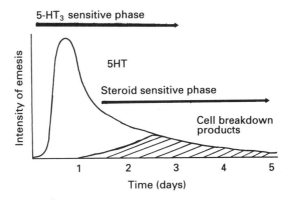

Figure 3.4 Acute and delayed vomiting after chemotherapy. Delayed vomiting is not so easily controlled as acute symptoms. It may be that 5-HT is the most important factor during the acute phase while other factors are becoming more influential over following days. (Modified from Andrews & Davis, 1993.)

factors which are more predominant at different times. It may be that better emetic control will be obtained when all factors are controlled from the outset.

In support of this hypothesis is the clinical finding that a combination of ondansetron and dexamethasone produces excellent control of cisplatin-induced emesis that was superior to that produced by metoclopramide plus dexamethasone plus diphenhydramine (see Figure 3.5). The superior control lasted for three days even though both groups received metoclopramide plus dexamethasone for days 2 to 4. (Italian Group for Antiemetic Research, 1992).

Although we do not know how steroids act to prevent emesis there is no doubt that they can enhance the efficacy of other antiemetics such as metoclopramide (Kris *et al.*, 1985b) and ondansetron (Bruntsch 1990; Smith *et al.*, 1990). Animal studies

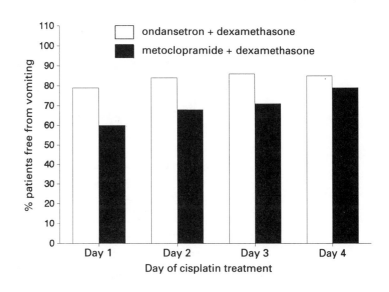

Figure 3.5 Ondansetron plus dexamethasone compared with metoclopramide plus dexamethasone in the control of cisplatin-induced vomiting. All patients received metoclopramide plus dexamethasone over days 2–5. (Data from Italian Group for Antiemetic Research, 1992.)

have shown that dexamethasone seems to have a synergistic action on 5-HT$_3$ receptor antagonist as dexamethasone plus ondansetron gave better control of emesis than the effect that would be expected from simply adding the individual effects of ondansetron and dexamethasone (Hawthorn & Cunningham, 1990).

As patients continue through several courses of chemotherapy some will develop anticipatory nausea and vomiting (ANV) – literally the mere anticipation of treatment will cause them to feel nauseous or they may even vomit.

Anticipatory nausea and vomiting

Anticipatory nausea and vomiting are thought to be conditioned responses (for review see Burish & Carey, 1986). Sights, smells or sounds which are present during a patient's treatment become associated with the treatment and specifically with the nausea and vomiting that follow treatment. After several cycles of therapy the patient only has to see, hear or smell the 'cue' and feelings of nausea ensue. In severe cases vomiting can occur. For some patients there is no one specific cue; just thinking about the treatment evokes this response.

Conditioned response

Classical conditioning is a process whereby two stimuli which originally elicit different responses in an organism come to elicit the same response. Perhaps the best known example is Pavlov's dogs, where ringing a bell as food was served conditioned the dogs to salivate on hearing the bell, whether food was present or not. In patients receiving chemotherapy the same phenomenon occurs. The chemotherapy is the unconditioned stimulus and the extraneous cue (for example sight of the nurse, sounds, smells) become paired with the unconditioned stimulus. These cues then become the conditioned stimulus. Nausea and vomiting are the conditioned response.

Common cues are the sight or smell of the hospital but quite often it can be the nurse who gives the chemotherapy. Many nurses will be wary of meeting their patients in the street because of the effect it can have. For some patients conjuring up a mental image of a chemotherapy session can precipitate anticipatory systems (Redd *et al.*, 1993). It has been shown that anticipatory nausea and vomiting can be long-lived phenomena.

Nerenz and colleagues (1986) have reported that in a group of patients recovering from Hodgkin's disease anticipatory symptoms were still present in over 50% of patients over two years later.

Incidence

Anticipatory nausea and vomiting has been documented in 30–65% of patients (Coons *et al.*, 1987), although anecdotal reports would suggest that it varies considerably with the type of cancer and for certain conditions, such as Hodgkin's lymphoma, it may be as high as 70–80% of patients.

Predisposing factors

The strongest predisposing factors for ANV are bad experiences of nausea and vomiting during early courses of chemotherapy (Andrykowski *et al.*, 1985; Dolgin *et al.*,1985, Nesse *et al.*, 1980). ANV is thus more likely to develop with the more emetogenic chemotherapy regimens. Other factors also contribute and we can outline the main ones. The experience of metallic taste or other unpleasant tastes during chemotherapy (Nerenz *et al.*, 1986). Patients who are anxious and/or hostile develop more ANV (Altmaier *et al.*, 1982; Morrow, 1984b; Andrykowski *et al.*, 1985; Ingle *et al.*, 1984).

Studies of the contribution of anxiety to the development of ANV have produced inconsistent results but this could be due to methodology. It is generally accepted, however, that anxiety is a facilitatory factor promoting the development of the conditioned response (for review see Cull, 1993).

On a physiological level there is evidence that anxiety is an important factor. Anxiety is associated with increased noradrenergic activity and clonidine, which reduces noradrenergic activity has been found to eliminate ANV in 50% of patients after a single cycle (Cull, 1993).

In one study patients who were younger, unmarried or on adjuvant CMF (cyclophosphamide, methotrexate, 5-fluorouracil) therapy were more prone to anticipatory nausea and vomiting (Fetting *et al.*, 1982). A susceptibility to motion sickness can predispose patients to anticipatory nausea and vomiting (Morrow, 1984b) and a fear of venepuncture also encourages the patient to develop anticipatory symptoms (Coons *et al.*, 1987). Infusions of long duration are more likely to induce anticipatory symptoms compared to short injections (Andrykowski *et al.*, 1985). Longer infusions may facilitate conditioning by increasing the exposure time to the clinic environment or may induce greater anxiety.The main factors are summarized in Table 3.6.

Table 3.6 Predisposing factors for anticipatory nausea and vomiting

- Poorly controlled nausea and vomiting during early course of treatment
- Prolonged nausea and vomiting after treatment
- Younger patients are more susceptible
- Anxiety or hostility
- Taste associated with drugs
- Susceptibility to motion sickness
- Fear of venepuncture

Development

It is primarily poorly controlled nausea and vomiting that cause the patient to develop anticipatory nausea and vomiting. For this reason the condition does not occur immediately and is usually seen only after several courses of chemotherapy. One author reported that anticipatory symptoms developed after three courses of therapy, and became more prevalent during cycles 4 and 5 (Nerenz *et al.*, 1986). As treatment progresses anticipatory nausea and vomiting, if untreated, will become worse.

Treatment

Anti-emetic drugs do not seem to control ANV (Morrow, 1992), although anxiolytics may help in reducing anxiety and thus prevent the condition developing. In psychological terms anticipatory nausea and vomiting is considered a conditioned response and as such responds to psychological interventions which break the association between the stimulus and the response (Burish *et al.*, 1987). Hypnosis, relaxation and systematic desensitization have all proved useful (Redd *et al.*, 1982; Morrow & Morrell, 1982) (see Chapter 5).

Psychological interventions, however, require a considerable amount of time and trained therapists. Unfortunately the old cliché is true – prevention is better than cure. Efficient control of emesis from the very first course of treatment will prevent the development of ANV.

3.5 Postoperative nausea and vomiting – PONV

The sickness occurring after surgery, postoperative nausea and vomiting (PONV), are caused by several factors which will be acting to stimulate the vomiting reflex before, during and after the surgical procedure.

Identifying the emetic stimulus is difficult. Emetic stimuli are additive and several factors occur during the pre- and peri-operative period which may predispose the patient to vomiting. Identification is confounded by the fact that a single event postoperatively may then precipitate actual vomiting but this is not the sole cause of the event.

The main factors which have been identified as influencing PONV are summarized in Table 3.7 and reviewed in more detail below.

Patient predisposition and demography

Gender

Women are two to three times more likely to suffer from PONV than men and the vomiting they experience is more severe (Burtles & Peckett, 1957; Bellville *et al.*, 1960). This is clearly related to female hormones since the incidence of PONV is comparable between the two sexes in children (Vance *et al.*, 1973) and increases in girls as the menarche is approached (Rita *et al.*, 1981), falling again after the menopause to levels similar to those found in males (Forrest *et al.*, 1990).

More recent studies have shown that the phase of the menstrual cycle will influence the intensity of symptoms (Beattie *et al.*, 1991). PONV are more pronounced and four times more likely to occur during the menses. Furthermore the anti-emetic

Table 3.7   Factors influencing PONV

- Patient predisposition and demography
- Operation site
- Drugs used in surgery – anaesthetics
                           – analgesics
                           – others
- Gastrointestinal disturbances – distension
                                  – decreased motility
- Visual/labyrinthine inputs
- Intubation of airways
- Pain/discomfort
- Hypotension
- Raised intracranial pressure
- Food in the stomach

used in one study, droperidol, was less effective in menstruating women than in those who were in a post-menstrual phase (Linblad *et al.*, 1990).

In support of the conclusion that these effects are due to high circulating levels of oestrogen is the observation that the addition of oestrogen to chemotherapy regimens for the treatment of breast cancer increases the incidence of nausea and vomiting (Benz *et al.*, 1987).

Age

The incidence of PONV is low in babies (Cohen *et al.*, 1990) and children under three years old (Rowley & Brown, 1982). Antiemetics are not routinely prescribed for the under fives except in cases of ear, nose and throat (ENT) surgery. Older children vomit more and pre-pubertal children (>3 < 12 years) were reported to be twice as likely to vomit as adults (Vance *et al.*, 1973). After puberty there is an increase in the incidence of emesis which is more pronounced in females (see above) and young females (puberty to 30 years) are probably the group most prone to PONV. The incidence of emesis remains fairly constant throughout adulthood but with advancing age there seems to be a correlation between increasing age and decreasing incidence of emesis (Burtles & Peckett, 1957; Bellville *et al.*, 1960).

Weight

It is usually accepted that obese patients experience more nausea and vomiting than thin patients (Smessaert *et al.*, 1959; Bellville *et al.*, 1960) (although these authors did not define 'obese' or 'thin'). This has been attributed to a larger mass of fat in which fat soluble anaesthetics can dissolve. It will take longer, therefore, for such anaesthetics to be fully metabolized and eliminated from the body. McKenzie and colleagues (1981) have reported more nausea and vomiting in heavier (>60 kg) patients when the period of anaesthesia lasted a mean of 25 minutes – not a long enough period, it has been suggested (Palazzo & Strunin, 1984a), for substantial differences in anaesthetic accumulation in fat to occur. One recent review article suggests that we do not have sufficient data to state that body mass index (a measure of the percentage body fat) *per se* is a predisposing factor to more PONV although many factors associated with being overweight may mean that these patients do experience more PONV (Lerman, 1992).

Susceptibility to motion sickness

It has been suggested that a susceptibility to motion sickness predisposes patients to PONV (Purkis, 1964). One study of women undergoing dilatation and curettage showed that 66% of patients who identified a cause thought that motion was the reason for their nausea and these patients were identified as having a susceptibility to motion sickness (Kamath *et al.*, 1990).

It has also been demonstrated that opioids can precipitate motion-induced nausea in conscious patients (Comroe & Dripps, 1948) the suggestion being that opioids sensitize the vestibular apparatus.

There is, however, considerable movement of the patient in the peri-operative period. The increased PONV seen in these patients may just be a reflection of their normal response to motion rather than increased sensitivity to the other contributory factors.

Anxiety

The precise contribution of anxiety to the aetiology of nausea and vomiting is not known. It is likely that the anxious patient will experience more PONV as has been seen in cancer patients. It is worth noting that patients undergoing investigative surgery or surgery for cancer may be particularly anxious. Some authors have suggested that more anxious patients swallow air and this contributes to gastrointestinal distension, exacerbating feelings of nausea and producing vomiting (Palazzo & Strunin, 1984a). These demographic factors are summarized in Table 3.8.

The influence of operation site

When the physiology of the emetic reflex is considered it is perhaps not surprising that high incidences of nausea and vomiting are associated with abdominal surgery (particularly gastrointestinal surgery) and procedures involving the ear, nose or throat (Palazzo & Strunin, 1984a; Cookson, 1986). Haumann and Foster (1963) noted high incidences of PONV after ENT or abdominal surgery and lowest incidences after head, neck and

---

Table 3.8 Demographic factors affecting PONV

- Gender – females are two to three times more likely to vomit than males
- Age – emesis increases after puberty but in adults decreases with increasing age
- Weight – obese patients vomit more than thin patients
- Susceptibility to motion sickness – susceptible patients vomit more after surgery
- Anxiety – anxious patients experience more PONV

chest operations. Such procedures will no doubt directly stimulate the afferent arm of the emetic reflex (see Chapter 2).

ENT and neurosurgery

This can stimulate the labyrinthine pathway of the emetic reflex. In addition there is an auricular branch of the vagus nerve which could be stimulated under such conditions.

The 'gag' reflex, as well as nausea and vomiting, can be elicited by pharyngeal stimulation; nausea and vomiting after paediatric tonsillectomy may be as high as 80% (van der Walt *et al.*, 1990). Vomiting can also be stimulated in these patients by the taste of blood or the presence of blood in the stomach.

Abdominal surgery

Abdominal surgery, especially that involving the viscera, is highly emetogenic. Bonica reported an incidence of nausea and vomiting of 70% in patients undergoing operations on the stomach, duodenum or gall bladder and 15% among abdominal wall procedures (Bonica *et al.*, 1958). The mechanisms could include direct stimulation of vagal pathways from the gut to the 'vomiting centre' or may also include release of substances from the gut which could stimulate vomiting. A candidate for this could be 5-HT. Abdominal surgery will usually result in post-operative ileus which can stimulate nausea and vomiting.

In particular patients undergoing laparoscopy experience particularly high incidence of PONV and this may be due to multiple abdominal stimuli – manipulation of the viscera and abdominal distension by gas.

Gynaecological surgery

This is associated with a high degree of PONV and dilatation and curettage will produce more postoperative emesis than curettage without dilation (Dundee *et al.*, 1962). Manipulation of the Fallopian tubes, for example in surgical sterilisation procedures, also seems to be associated with a high incidence of nausea and vomiting.

Adenotonsillectomy

Adenotonsillectomy is associated with a high incidence of PONV (36–76%). This is thought to be due to the irritant effect of blood on oesophageal chemoreceptors, direct stimulations of the trigeminal nerve and the fact that opioids are commonly used (Lerman, 1992).

Strabismus surgery

Strabismus surgery is associated with a high degree of nausea and vomiting (White & Schafer, 1987). Many of the patients undergoing this type of surgery are children (who are prone to vomiting) and it is important that the delicate surgery is not disrupted. Strabismus surgery represents, therefore, a particularly high-risk group.

Influence of anaesthetics

Local anaesthetics

Local anaesthetics generally are not associated with nausea and vomiting.

Spinal anaesthesia

Spinal anaesthesia causes nausea and vomiting but a large component of this effect is likely to be the hypotension subsequent to blocking blood pressure regulatory mechanisms. Datta and colleagues (1982) showed that the incidence of nausea and vomiting was 66% in patients with spinal anaesthesia and some degree of hypotension but this was reduced to 10% if the hypotension was treated with intravenous ephedrine. Other studies have also demonstrated that falls in systolic pressure below 80 mm Hg during spinal anaesthesia can increase emesis significantly (Crocker & Vandam, 1959; Ratra *et al.*, 1972).

It has been suggested that some degree of hypoxia at the vomiting centre is responsible for nausea and vomiting during spinal anaesthesia (Ratra *et al.*, 1972). These authors reported a decreased incidence of emesis when 100% oxygen was employed, despite low systolic pressures.

Epidural anaesthesia generally produces less hypotension than spinal anaesthesia.

If the patient is experiencing discomfort, pain or anxiety because they are conscious this can increase the amount of nausea and vomiting.

Inhalation anaesthetics

Early inhalation anaesthetics were notorious for their emetic action, ether being a particular culprit, causing nausea and vomiting in up to 82% of patients (Knapp & Beecher, 1956).

The advent of inhalation agents such as cyclopropane and halothane, which superseded ether, radically changed this picture as these agents showed much lower incidences of nausea and vomiting. Recently cyclopropane has been withdrawn as its explosive properties present a hazard in the operating theatre.

Halothane is associated with a low level of postoperative vomiting – the incidence of emesis during the first six hours after anaesthesia has been reported as only 5% (Haumann & Foster, 1963).

Isoflurane, despite being a chemical related to, and sharing many of the irritant properties of, ether has a similar emetic profile to halothane (McAteer *et al.*, 1986). Enflurane is similarly associated with a low incidence of nausea and vomiting (Gaskey *et al.*, 1986).

The commonly used anaesthetic gas nitrous oxide has perhaps been most widely investigated for emetic activity. Nitrous oxide has been shown to have a direct emetic action as it induces nausea in volunteers in a concentration dependant manner (Parkhouse *et al.*, 1960). The incidence of nausea increased as the nitrous oxide concentration was raised from 20% to 40%.

The contribution of nitrous oxide to the overall incidence of PONV is controversial. Nitrous oxide has been claimed to increase PONV (Alexander *et al.*, 1984; Lonie & Harper, 1986) while in other studies the omission of nitrous oxide from iso-flurane or enflurane anaesthesia did not affect the incidence of postoperative vomiting (Korttila *et al.*, 1987; Muir *et al.*, 1987; Melnik & Johnson, 1987; Hovorka *et al.*, 1989).

It may be that the length of exposure to this gas influences the incidence of postoperative vomiting (Bodman *et al.*, 1960; Morrison *et al.*, 1968). One study has concluded that the dura-tion of anaesthesia (opioid/nitrous oxide/relaxant) was unim-portant (Kvisselgaard, 1958).

Nitrous oxide probably acts through central and peripheral mechanisms (Palazzo & Strunin, 1984a) although it has been claimed that it does not stimulate the 'vomiting centre' (Adriani *et al.*, 1961).

It has been suggested that nitrous oxide interacts with the endogenous opioid system and thus shares some of the emetic actions of opioids (Gillman, 1985).

Many of the emetic actions of nitrous oxide have been ascribed to the physical effects of the gas.

Physical effects of inhalation agents

Physical problems associated with the presence of gases such as nitrous oxide are diffusion into the middle ear where excess pressure perturbs the vestibular apparatus and thereby stimu-lates vomiting (Davis *et al.*, 1979).

Nitrous oxide may also diffuse into the stomach and colon, causing distension which may stimulate the emetic reflex and certainly leads to abdominal discomfort during the post-operative period (Palazzo & Strunin, 1984a). This is a slow process and would probably only make a significant contribution to PONV after long periods of exposure. Accumulation of anaesthetic would be exacerbated by the fact that both belching and elimination of gas as flatus are inhibited in the anaesthetized patient.

Introduction of gas into the gastrointestinal tract during manual ventilation with a mask may occur, especially if the anaesthetist is inexperienced (Hovorka *et al.*, 1990). The differences in the emetic action of nitrous oxide discussed above may therefore be due, in part, to its more careful use by some anaesthetists (Palazzo & Strunin, 1984a).

Intravenous anaesthetics

Several studies have compared inhalational with intravenous agents. While there are obviously differences between the compounds themselves as well as in the route of administration, the overall conclusion seems to be that intravenous anaesthetic agents are less emetogenic than inhalational agents. Thus an intravenous regimen of propofol and alfentanil has been demonstrated to be associated with significantly less nausea and vomiting than nitrous oxide and enflurane in women undergoing minor gynaecological surgery (Raftery & Sherry, 1992). A similar study showed that women anaesthetized with propofol alone fared better in terms of PONV than either the propofol/nitrous oxide group or the propofol/nitrous oxide/enflurane group (Gunwardene & White, 1988). Fewer children undergoing strabismus surgery suffered postoperative vomiting after propofol/fentanyl anaesthesia than after thiopentone/halothane (Larsson *et al.*, 1992).

One author has suggested that intravenous anaesthetics fall into two groups. Those with a slow and smooth recovery profile tend to be associated with a low incidence of nausea and vomiting – for example thiopentone. Whereas those associated with rapid recovery characteristics and a high degree of excitatory effects produce more PONV – for example ketamine (Clarke, 1984).

Influence of analgesics

For some minor surgery analgesics comprise a large part of the anaesthetic procedure and analgesics with or without anxiolytics form part of the pre-medication for major surgery. Analgesics may also be given during surgery and/or on recovery. Morphine, the 'foundation stone analgesic' of surgical anaesthesia, is particularly notorious for its emetic action.

Morphine is thought to depress the 'vomiting centre' but stimulates the CTZ. The CTZ contains a high density of μ opioid receptors (Leslie, 1985). Thus it could cause emesis directly.

Other actions of morphine include a slowing of gastric emptying and decrease in gastric motility, which may add to feelings of nausea. Morphine slows colonic transport, causing constipation which, as well as producing discomfort, can cause nausea and vomiting in some patients. The effects of morphine on gastric emptying are prolonged and can extend into the postoperative period. The decreased emptying is associated with an increased gastric tone. The tension in the gastric wall is, therefore, higher than it would be in the absence of morphine. When the patient tries to take water or food during the postoperative period the combined effects of decreased emptying and increased gastric tone cause a greater stimulation of the mechanoreceptors than would normally occur and this can trigger feelings of nausea or vomiting (Andrews, 1992).

The emetic activity of morphine is dose related. The dose administered should, therefore, be kept to the minimum required for efficient analgesia as increasing doses above this will not provide better pain relief but will exacerbate vomiting (Clarke, 1991).

When given by epidural administration morphine causes nausea and vomiting in up to five times more patients than when given intravenously (Bromage *et al.*, 1982; Cousins & Mather, 1984).

Both morphine and pethidine (meperidine) appear to increase the sensitivity of the labyrinthine apparatus and the incidence of vomiting after morphine is increased in ambulatory compared with recumbent patients (Purkis 1964; Riding, 1975).

In attempts to reduce the amount of postoperative vomiting other opioids have been used. Papaveretum is a mixture of opium alkaloids standardized to contain 50% morphine (equivalent to 53% morphine sulphate). However, there is no evidence that its use is accompanied by less sickness than seen with morphine sulphate (Loan *et al.*, 1966). One of the components of papaveretum, noscopine, is thought to be associated with teratogenic effects. For this reason papaveretum has generally been replaced by proprietary alkaloid mixtures that have recently been reformulated and no longer contain noscopine.

Pethidine may appear to cause less emesis but this effect is more likely to be due to the shorter half-life of pethidine; its emetic action is waning by one hour after administration whereas the emetic action of morphine continues for at least six hours (Dundee *et al.*, 1965).

The practice of giving these opioids pre-operatively has been discontinued almost entirely in the USA and is decreasing in the UK although they are still widely used pre- and post-operatively. Concomitantly the use of pre-operative benzodiazepines is increasing.

Fentanyl is a relatively new opiate derivative widely used in gynaecological and cardiac surgery. It can be highly emetogenic and several studies have demonstrated that the addition of fentanyl to the anaesthetic regimen increases the amount of nausea and vomiting (Hackett *et al.*, 1982; Melnick *et al.*, 1984; Rising *et al.*, 1985; Gaskey *et al.*, 1986).

Closely related analgesics alfentanil and sufentanil are more lipid soluble but have similar emetic profiles.

Other drugs used in surgery

Hyoscine and atropine are given before surgery for their anti-sialagogue (inhibition of saliva secretion) activity. Both also have anti-emetic activity. Hyoscine is most commonly encountered as an anti-emetic for travel (motion) sickness. As such it will be useful in counteracting the labyrinthine inputs.

One study carefully documented the anti-emetic action of atropine when combined with the emetic morphine (Riding, 1960). Using large patient groups of women undergoing curettage under thiopentone, nitrous oxide/oxygen, he showed that morphine was emetic in a dose related manner and this could be reduced in a dose related fashion by atropine.

Muscle relaxants are generally not thought to be emetic. Anxiolytics such as benzodiazepines are not emetic. Some especially lorazepam have anti-emetic and amnesic effects (Laszlo *et al.*, 1985), both of which are beneficial to the surgical patient.

The reversal agent neostigmine is emetic. This may be because it stimulates vagal activity causing violent gut motility. Such vagal activation can result in cardiac disturbances, causing profound bradycardia, as well as nausea and vomiting. For this reason atropine or glycopyrrolate are usually given with neostigmine, to block the vagal activation.

In one study using neostigmine/atropine reversal the incidence of nausea was 68% in the reversal group compared with 32% in the no reversal group. Vomiting was 47% compared with 11% respectively (King *et al.*, 1988). The anti-emetic activity of atropine alone would not appear sufficient to counteract the action of neostigmine.

Gastrointestinal disturbances

There are several ways in which surgery can perturb gastro-intestinal function and cause or intensify PONV. Obviously any manipulation of the gut during surgery will stimulate mechanoreceptors and maybe chemoreceptors in the gut. Manipulation may also cause a release of 5-HT from the enterochromaffin cells which would stimulate the emetic reflex.

Surgery will disrupt gastrointestinal motility. A cessation of gastrointestinal motility is a common effect of anaesthesia. This has usually been ascribed to increases in sympathetic activity.

Anaesthetics can reduce the tone of the lower oesophageal sphincter (LOS). This may not actually stimulate emesis but decreased LOS pressure means that the patient is more likely to experience regurgitation with the attendant risk of aspiration (Brock-Utne *et al.*, 1978).

Gastrointestinal stasis will also mean that gut secretions and swallowed saliva will accumulate. Such secretions and maybe also gas will cause distension which is a known emetic stimulus.

Visual/ labyrinthine effects

Stimulation of the labyrinthine pathway stimulates emesis. There is considerable stimulation of the ear due to the movement associated with surgery (from bed to trolley to operating table to trolley to bed) which can produce feelings of nausea. Patients may find being wheeled on a trolley while lying down particularly disorienting.

Being sat up after recovery often stimulates emesis. This may be a combination of labyrinthine stimulation and the fall in blood pressure that will occur on sitting up or standing.

Intubation of airways

As an airway or endotracheal tube is inserted through the mouth as part of surgical and other procedures it is inevitable that there will be stimulation of the pharynx. This can activate the emetic reflex (see Chapter 2). The airway should be inserted by a skilled person and removed before the gag reflex is re-established to minimize vomiting (Palazzo & Strunin, 1984b).

Suction can also stimulate pharyngeal pathways and pharyngeal suction is best done before reversal of muscle relaxation (Palazzo & Strunin, 1984b).

Pain

Pain is a stimulus known to contribute to nausea and vomiting. Visceral or pelvic pain in the postoperative period is a common cause of nausea (Parkhouse, 1963).

There is some evidence which suggests that pain is associated more with nausea rather than frank vomiting. Thus one study of the postoperative period demonstrated that 10% of patients had pain without nausea whereas 58% had pain accompanied by nausea (Andersen & Krohg, 1976). Furthermore, excessive doses of naloxone (an opioid antagonist) caused the return of both pain and nausea and vomiting (Adriani *et al.*, 1961).

Although opioids are in themselves emetic they should not be withheld for treating pain on this basis. Andersen & Krohg (1976) showed that pain and nausea was reduced in 80% of episodes whereas the opioid induced nausea in only 3.4% of cases.

Hypotension

Anaesthetics and blood loss during surgical procedures give rise to hypotension. This is not usually a problem as blood pressure regulatory mechanisms recover as the patient wakes. However if blood pressure remains low or if spinal anaesthesia is causing hypotension, then nausea and vomiting can occur. Postural hypotension can occur when a recumbent patient stands up for the first time and this may precipitate feelings of nausea.

Raised intracranial pressure

As stated earlier, raised intracranial pressure (ICP) is associated with vomiting especially sudden, forceful vomiting unheralded by feelings of nausea. Neurosurgery can result in raised intracranial pressure. Halothane, enflurane and ketamine all cause elevations of intracranial pressure via vasodilatory actions on the cerebral blood vessels. This is a potential source of nausea. In most circumstances this is probably a small risk factor but in some cases, e.g. neurosurgery, where raised ICP is likely to be occurring due to the surgery, it must be considered. Isoflurane has less action in raising ICP and is therefore used in neurosurgical procedures. Barbiturates (thiopentone, pentobarbitone) lower intracranial pressure and can be used to counteract the action of the anaesthetics (Davson *et al.*, 1987).

Food in the stomach

For elective surgery the patient is always fasted prior to surgery as food in the stomach is known to stimulate vomiting both during induction and recovery. Stomach emptying takes an average of six hours for solid food and four hours for fluids (Carrie & Simpson, 1988) but patients are often 'nil-by-mouth' for longer periods.

For surgical emergencies prior fasting is obviously not possible. Some anaesthetists use gastrokinetic agents (those which increase gastric motility) such as metoclopramide to promote

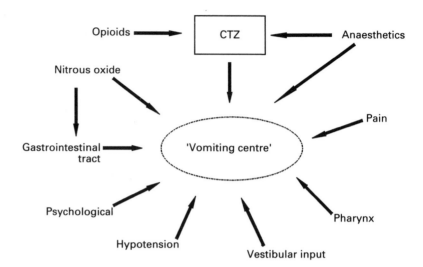

Figure 3.6 Factors influencing PONV.

gastric emptying (Howarth *et al.*, 1969) or gastric aspiration is employed. These measures are not always efficient and close monitoring of such patients is essential.

A rapid induction phase accompanied by cricoid pressure (Sellick's manoeuvre) is the most common method for avoiding regurgitation of stomach contents during induction of anaesthesia (Palazzo & Strunin, 1984b).

Postoperatively gastrointestinal distension (either because of food, secretions or gas) may be a problem. In these circumstances gastric decompression using a tube has proved useful (Smessaert *et al.*, 1959).

The main factors influencing PONV are summarized in Figure 3.6.

3.6 Pregnancy sickness

It is well known that the majority of pregnant women will experience some nausea and/or vomiting during their pregnancy that generally decreases as the pregnancy progresses. Although it is commonly called 'morning sickness' this is a misnomer as it is clear that the nausea and/or vomiting are not restricted to the morning. Despite the prevalence of this condition and the fact that we have known of its existence for many years – the earliest description written on papyrus has been dated around 2000 BC (see Andrews & Whitehead, 1990) – little is known for certain about its aetiology. Associated with pregnancy sickness is the more serious condition of *hyperemesis gravidarum* which is characterized by intractable nausea and vomiting throughout the pregnancy which can give rise to poor nutrition and electrolyte imbalance.

Incidence of pregnancy sickness

A large (1000 subjects) survey of pregnant women in South London, showed that 85% of pregnant women suffered from nausea and 52% from vomiting (Whitehead *et al.*, 1992). Most women (73%) were suffering from nausea within six weeks of the last menstrual period (LMP), nearly half of these reporting symptoms within four weeks. Often the feelings of nausea are a signal to a woman that she may be pregnant. Generally the earlier the symptoms appear the more frequent they tended to be. Pregnancy sickness tends to subside and disappear around 14–18 weeks of gestation, although a small percentage of patients have mild symptoms to the end of their pregnancy. Later in the pregnancy direct effects of the growing fetus on the mother's gastrointestinal tract may be responsible for symptoms (see below).

Hyperemesis gravidarum is a much rarer condition occurring in around 1:1000 pregnancies.

Causes of pregnancy sickness

Psychological explanations have been sought for pregnancy sickness but studies have been unable to give any consistent correlations of nausea and vomiting with how planned or wanted the pregnancy was. Symptoms could not be correlated with whether the pregnant woman was single or co-habiting or with how many people they felt they could count on for support (Whitehead *et al.*, 1992).

Hormones have been investigated as perhaps the most obvious culprits for inducing pregnancy sickness. However, no consistent differences in the circulating levels of oestrogens, progestagens, androgens or cortisol can be observed in serial blood samples from women experiencing sickness compared with those who were not (Jarnfelt-Samsioe, 1987). It is even more tempting to ascribe pregnancy sickness to human chorionic gonadotrophin (hCG) as this hormone rises sharply in early pregnancy, peaks between eight and ten weeks gestation and falls again to lower levels around weeks 14–18; a time course that parallels the incidence of emetic symptoms. However, studies have generally been unable to show any association between hCG levels and emesis with reports quoting lower, similar or higher levels of hCG in symptomatic and non-symptomatic pregnancies. Even in subjects with hydatiform mole, where levels of hCG are extremely high, no correlation could be found between hormone levels and the incidence or severity of nausea and vomiting (Soules *et al.*, 1980).

The lack of any connection between these hormones and the emetic symptoms may be due to the fact that individual women have very different thresholds for the effects of hormones, or the nausea and vomiting could be the result of subtle interactions between the various hormones and it may be the ratio of hormones rather than their absolute levels that stimulate the emetic reflex. In support of these hypotheses are the observations that the majority of women who experience sickness with the contraceptive pill (91%) develop pregnancy sickness – denoting their low individual threshold – and that the progesterone only pill causes far fewer symptoms of nausea and vomiting (see Andrews & Whitehead, 1990).

One report has shown a correlation between degree of activation of the thyroid gland and suppression of TSH secretion and the incidence and severity of pregnancy sickness (Mori *et al.*, 1988).

Steroid hormones secreted during pregnancy can have effects on the gastrointestinal system including an inhibitory action on the smooth muscle of the gut, decreased lower oesophageal sphincter pressure (Van Thiez *et al.*, 1977) and decreased gastric emptying with increased gut transit times (Lawson *et al.*, 1985).

3.7 Vomiting due to eating disorders

The vomiting due to eating disorders rarely has an organic cause and is usually self-induced by the patient. There are several ways in which patients make themselves vomit but the most common are by pharyngeal stimulation – achieved by the patient putting the fingers down the throat or by using something like a toothbrush to stimulate the pharynx. Sometimes the patients's food consumption has been so large that the mechanical distension of the stomach is enough to produce vomiting.

These eating disorders are more prevalent in women than men and have a higher incidence in teenagers and young adults (<30 years). Although these disorders usually start with the patient's desire to be slim, they are generally symptomatic of a deeper psychological problem and the patient invariably needs some degree of psychological or psychiatric help.

Anorexia nervosa　Colloquially called the 'slimmer's disease', this commonly starts with strict dieting and a desire to become very slim and stay so. Frequently preoccupied with food, the patient is also obsessed by her own body image. Weight loss frequently goes past the fashionably thin to an emaciated state. The patient becomes tired and weak and lanugo hair (fine downy hair) grows on the body. The anorexic tries to avoid food in an obsessive way but will sometime 'binge' – eat a huge amount – and then make herself sick. Large amounts of laxatives are also used to try and remove the offending food.

Bulimia nervosa　This closely related condition is also characterized by an obsession with food. Bulimics are not necessarily so emaciated and undernourished as anorexics. Nevertheless, their physical and psychological health is impaired (Norman & Herzog, 1986). They tend to eat large amounts of food and make themselves vomit on a regular basis.

The study and treatment of these eating disorders is a vast topic, beyond the scope of this book. There is much debate as to the aetiology of these conditions, but many authorities tend towards the view that young girls with anorexia are having difficulty in growing up and accepting their femininity and sexuality. Their thinness is an expression of trying to retain a childlike shape and as severe weight loss affects gonadotrophic and ovarian function there is a concomitant amenorrhoea (cessation of periods) which reinforces the childlike body image that patient is seeking.

Electrolyte imbalance becomes quite severe and the metabolic disturbances consequent to prolonged vomiting can be life-threatening.

Treatment of anorexia and bulimia require medical supervision of the patient's physical condition as well as psychiatric help. Psychological treatment is generally thought to have better long-term effects than drug treatments, at least for bulimia (Treasure *et al.*, 1994). There is increasing interest in self-directed manuals for treating such conditions which not only assist the patient in gaining a sense of control and mastering their own illness but also make the treatment more widely available and less restricted to highly specialized units (Treasure *et al.*, 1994).

Summary of Chapter 3

- Vomiting in babies may be due to a congenital defect, infection, disease or allergy to formula milk.
- Projectile vomiting may be indicative of pyloric stenosis.
- Motion sickness is due to a 'mis-match' between visual and labyrinthine information.
- Gastrointestinal diseases and obstruction can cause nausea and vomiting.
- Several diseases and some drugs cause nausea and vomiting.
- Not every cancer patient will be sick; personal characteristics can influence the susceptibility of a patient to treatment-induced nausea and vomiting.
- Radiotherapy is generally less emetogenic than chemotherapy. The amount of vomiting in response to chemotherapy depends on the drugs used.
- The latency to feeling nauseous or vomiting will depend on the treatment given.
- Vomiting may be acute, delayed or anticipatory.
- PONV is caused by a variety of factors acting alone or in concert.
- Patient characteristics, analgesics, anaesthetics, other drugs, and the operation site are the most important determining factors.
- Females and younger adults are most prone to PONV.
- Inhalational agents are generally more emetic than intravenous agents.
- Opioids and opioid derivatives are emetogenic but should not be withheld on this basis.
- Surgery involving the ears, nose and throat, abdominal, gynaecological and paediatric strabismus procedures are the most emetic.
- Other factors influencing the incidence of PONV include the physical effects of gases, raised intracranial pressure, labyrinthine effects, intubation of airways, pain, hypotension and the presence of food in the stomach.
- Careful attention to these factors will aid in controlling PONV.
- Pregnancy sickness is quite common and not detrimental to the outcome of the pregnancy.

- The causes of pregnancy sickness are not fully understood.
- Vomiting due to eating disorders rarely has an organic cause.
- Patients with eating disorders need psychological or psychiatric support.

1. Pyloric stenosis in babies:

   TRUE   FALSE

   (a) is characterized by projectile vomiting
   (b) does not occur during the first year of life
   (c) can be corrected by surgery
   (d) is due to allergy to milk formula

2. Rate the following statements as true or false:

   (a) moving scenery can make a person feel sick even if they are standing still
   (b) closing your eyes when on board ship will help relieve seasickness
   (c) motion sickness does not predispose to chemotherapy-induced nausea and vomiting

3. Nausea and vomiting can be caused by:

   (a) antibiotics
   (b) Ménière's disease
   (c) hypocalcaemia
   (d) urinary tract infections

4. Vomiting a large amount of undigested food is a symptom of:

   (a) enlarged liver
   (b) indigestion
   (c) gastrointestinal obstruction
   (d) bony metastases

5. Pregnancy sickness: TRUE   FALSE

   (a) is more common in unplanned
       pregnancies
   (b) occurs in around 25% of pregnancies
   (c) subsides around 14–18 weeks of
       pregnancy
   (d) is due to high levels of hCG
   (e) is detrimental to the pregnancy

6. Radiation is unlikely to induce emesis if
   the dose is kept below (mark one box
   with a tick):

   (a) 2 Gy
   (b) 5 Gy
   (c) 10 Gy
   (d) 20 Gy

7. Indicate with a tick those factors
   considered important in the emetic
   response to radiotherapy:

   (a) age
   (b) gender
   (c) site of irradiation
   (d) age of the radiotherapy apparatus
   (e) high alcohol intake

8. Chemotherapy-induced vomiting is more
   prevalent in:

   (a) women than men
   (b) patients with a history of high
       alcohol intake
   (c) patients receiving chemotherapy for
       the first time compared with those on
       a second or third course of therapy
   (d) anxious patients
   (e) elderly patients

9. Rank the following drugs in order of
   emetic potential:
   (1 = most emetic, 4 = least emetic)   TRUE   FALSE

   (a) bleomycin (iv)
   (b) cisplatin (iv)
   (c) cyclophosphamide (iv)
   (d) epirubicin (iv)

10. Are the following statements true or
    false?

    (a) all patients will respond the same to
        every course of therapy provided
        their treatment drugs are not changed
    (b) if chemotherapy is repeated on
        consecutive days the amount of
        nausea and vomiting increases daily
    (c) the route of administration can affect
        the emetic potential of a cytotoxic
        drug

11. Anticipatory nausea and vomiting are
    more common:

    (a) after the third cycle than after the
        first cycle of therapy
    (b) in patients who do not have delayed
        emesis
    (c) in patients who are not sick on their
        first course of therapy

12. Delayed nausea and vomiting:

    (a) do not occur if the patient is not sick
        on the day of treatment
    (b) most commonly occur with
        cisplatin, ifosfamide and
        cyclophosphamide
    (c) need lower doses of anti-emetics to
        control it than acute emesis
    (d) start 12 hours after chemotherapy

13. Anti-emetic drugs for chemo- and
    radiotherapy-induced vomiting may be
    antagonists at:　　　　　　　　　　　　TRUE　FALSE

    (a) dopamine receptors
    (b) histamine receptors
    (c) 5-hydroxytrypamine (serotonin)
        receptors
    (d) noradrenaline receptors

14. Mark with a tick the two patients who are
    most likely to vomit after their operation:

    (a) a 35 year old woman undergoing
        dilatation and curettage
    (b) a 2 year old boy having an operation
        on his leg
    (c) a menstruating woman undergoing
        ENT surgery
    (d) a 50 year old man having a hernia
        repair

15. Place the following in order of
    emetogenic potential
    (1 = most emetic; 4 = least emetic)

    (a) propofol
    (b) ether
    (c) halothane
    (d) nitrous oxide

16. The emetic action of morphine is:

    (a) due to stimulation of the CTZ
    (b) accompanied by slowed colonic
        transit time
    (c) due to increased gastric motility
    (d) dose related
    (e) less when the morphine is given by
        epidural rather than intravenous
        route

17. Rate the following statements as true
    or false:

	TRUE	FALSE
(a) muscle relaxants are not emetogenic		
(b) neostigmine does not cause emesis		
(c) atropine increases salivation		
(d) inhalational agents are more emetogenic than intravenous		

CHAPTER 4: ANTI-EMETIC DRUGS

Anti-emetics comprise a rather pharmacologically diverse group of drugs. Most were not developed as anti-emetics, but were borrowed from other areas of medicine when found to have anti-emetic properties. Sometimes we do not understand how these drugs are acting to control emesis (e.g. steroids). For other drugs several pharmacological actions have been identified and it is not always clear which actions confer anti-emetic activity on the compound. For example, a common side-effect of many anti-emetics is that they produce sedation in the patient. Their anti-emetic activity may in fact be due to this sedation as the patient may well sleep through periods of nausea and be less distressed. Although under other circumstances sedation may be undesirable.

It is only recently, with the understanding of the role of 5-HT in emesis and the development of selective 5-HT$_3$ receptor antagonists that we have seen drugs specifically designed as anti-emetics (see Chapter 2). However, even these drugs are not universal anti-emetics and are not effective in every situation.

This chapter considers the main classes of anti-emetic drugs and the commonly encountered examples. They are summarized in Table 4.1.

The majority of currently available anti-emetics are dopamine receptor antagonists, even if they have other actions. Thus substituted benzamides, butyrophenones, substituted butyrophenones and phenothiazines are all dopamine antagonists. The reasons why dopamine receptor antagonists have been used so widely as anti-emetics were outlined in Chapter 2, but are worth re-iterating.

First, dopamine is involved in the control of gastric motility and dopamine receptor antagonists are used in a variety of gastrointestinal disorders. They generally increase peristalsis and thus decrease reflux; agents such as metoclopramide and domperidone are used to facilitate gastric emptying.

Second, there are dopamine receptors in the CTZ and in the NTS, which may be involved in the vomiting reflex (see Chapter 2). Third, apomorphine, a dopamine agonist, is also a powerful emetic and this emetic action can be prevented by dopamine

Table 4.1 The main classes of anti-emetic drugs

Anticholinergics	Hyoscine
	Atropine
Antihistamines	Diphenhydramine
	Cinnarizine
	Dimenhydrinate
	Meclozine
	Promethazine
	Cyclizine
Butyrophenones	Haloperidol
	Droperidol
Substituted butyrophenone	Domperidone
Phenothiazines	Prochlorperazine
	Chlorpromazine
	Perphenazine
Corticosteroids	Dexamethasone
	Methylprednisolone
Benzodiazepines	Lorazepam
Cannabinoids	Tetrahydro-cannabinol (THC)
	Nabilone
Substituted benzamides	Metoclopramide
5-HT$_3$ receptor antagonists	Ondansetron
	Granisetron
	Tropisetron

receptor antagonists. This led to the belief that all emesis could be controlled by dopamine antagonists, which is not true. Although anti-dopaminergic compounds are effective in controlling the vomiting produced by cytotoxic drugs of low emetogenic potential, they are less effective against highly emetogenic drug regimens, especially cisplatin. The use of metoclopramide at high doses provided the clue that it was probably antagonism of 5-HT at the 3 receptor which was more important in these cases. This is explained in greater detail in Chapter 2.

4.1 Side-effects of dopamine antagonists

Dopamine has many actions in the central nervous system (CNS) and the use of dopamine receptor antagonists unfortunately can affect these actions resulting in a variety of undesirable side effects, notably hypotension, sedation, agitation and a constellation of symptoms known as extrapyramidal reactions (EPRs).

The onset of EPRs often start with the feeling that the tongue is swelling up inside the mouth (it isn't) and some patients find their back teeth grinding and their jaw locks. Most patients experience restlessness, akathisia (involuntary shaking of the limbs), oculogyric crises (spasm of the muscles controlling eyeball movement) and torticollis (spasm of neck and facial muscles causing twisting of the head). The more severe disturbances of movement are sometimes called acute dystonic reactions; generally this term does not include restlessness.

Extrapyramidal reactions are particularly problematic (DiSilva et al., 1973). These occur more frequently in children and young adults (Bateman et al., 1989) and are exacerbated if dopamine receptor antagonists are given on consecutive days. Anecdotally, middle-aged females seem to suffer more than other groups from restlessness and agitation. As several regimens for paediatric malignancies utilize chemotherapy on a daily dosing schedule, particular care must be taken when choosing anti-emetics for this patient group.

Extrapyramidal reactions (EPR)
The extrapyramidal system of the brain is a complex neuronal network extending from the cortex to the medulla. Descending spinal pathways originate in the extrapyramidal system which influence voluntary motor activity and muscle tone.

Much of the activity of the extrapyramidal tract involves dopaminergic pathways. Therefore a disturbance of normal dopaminergic transmission causes an inability to co-ordinate voluntary movement, alterations in muscle tone and the occurrence of involuntary movements. These are known as extrapyramidal reactions (EPRs).

The most severe cases of extrapyramidal disturbances are seen in Parkinson's disease, but similar problems are caused by the administration of dopamine receptor antagonists.

4.2 Pharmacological action and clinical use of the common anti-emetic drugs

This section outlines the clinical use of the major anti-emetic agents. For full information on any of the drugs mentioned here the manufacturers' data sheets should always be consulted.

Anticholinergics

Isolated from the plant *Belladonna* (deadly nightshade) the anticholinergic drugs have been known to man for centuries. Anticholinergic drugs are thought to have a direct depressant action on the vomiting centre and an antispasmodic action on the gut. Hyoscine (scopolamine) is used in irritable bowel syndrome. Both hyoscine and atropine are used to control motion sickness and are frequently encountered in surgery as part of the pre-medication regimen where their antisialogogue and anti-emetic properties are useful. Hyoscine is reported to be the more effective of the two (Clarke, 1984).

Anticholinergics are not usually used for radio- or chemotherapy-induced nausea and vomiting (Hogan, 1990).

Both drugs are available as tablets and injections. Recently transdermal patches of hyoscine have been developed. They are particularly useful for travel sickness and have been used prophylactically in surgery. One study demonstrated that the patches significantly reduced PONV when compared with placebo in women undergoing gynaecological surgery (Loper *et al.*, 1989).

All anticholinergic agents produce dilation of the pupils and dry mouth. Drowsiness and urinary retention are common side-effects.

Hyoscine is not usually given to patients over 65 years of age as it can cause confusion, drowsiness, disorientation, dizziness and visual hallucinations in these patients. In cases where this so-called 'central cholinergic syndrome' might occur atropine would be used.

Antihistamines

First introduced in 1944 these drugs comprise a heterogeneous group of agents. They antagonize the action of histamine at the H_1 receptor. The most common are dimenhydrinate, cyclizine, cinnarizine, meclozine, promethazine and diphenhydramine. These preparations are excellent for treating travel sickness but have a major drawback in causing sedation. Most OTC (over the counter) preparations for travel sickness are antihistamines. They are only poorly effective in controlling chemotherapy-induced nausea and vomiting but are often included in anti-emetic cocktails. In these cases it is likely that their main contribution is in sedating the patient.

In the surgical situation cyclizine, a piperazine derivative, is the most extensively used antihistamine. It is as effective as perphenazine when used prophylactically and can also control established vomiting (Dundee *et al.*, 1975), although it has a short duration of action (four hours).

Butyrophenones   The butyrophenones haloperidol and droperidol are dopamine receptor antagonists thought to act on dopamine receptors in the CTZ. They can act centrally (their initial use was psychiatric for treating schizophrenia) which results in a variety of EPRs. Furthermore large doses of droperidol can cause cardiovascular and sedative effects (Korttila *et al.*, 1979).

In four uncontrolled studies, haloperidol and droperidol were shown to be useful anti-emetics against a variety of chemotherapy regimens (see Donovitz *et al.*, 1984). Haloperidol is less effective than metoclopramide (Grunberg *et al.*,1984). Although not widely used in oncology units as a single agent, haloperidol is often employed in combination therapy and is more widely used in palliative care (see below).

Intravenous droperidol has been shown to be effective in treating PONV (Patton *et al.*, 1974; Iwamoto & Schwartz, 1978; Korttila *et al.*, 1979; Rita *et al.*, 1981; Santos & Datta, 1984). Droperidol 5 mg (intra muscular) is slower in onset than haloperidol 2 mg (Loeser *et al.*, 1979) and has a shorter half-life. Postoperative recovery from anaesthesia can be significantly delayed by droperidol (Rowbotham, 1992). Despite these facts droperidol is more widely used than haloperidol. Droperidol is also effective for paediatric patients (Lerman *et al.*, 1986), although in some similar studies emesis was only controlled in around 30–40% of children.

This level of control was reported as ineffective in two studies (Friesen & Lockhart, 1992; Yentis & Bissonnette, 1992), while a third reported this level of control as acceptable (Lin et al., 1992). All these studies evaluated children undergoing strabismus surgery; given the delicacy of the surgery and the distress the children would suffer, a control level of 30% would probably be considered unacceptable by most anaesthetists.

A further study has shown the efficacy of droperidol to be decreased in women who were actively menstruating at the time of surgery (Linblad *et al.*, 1990).

Substituted butyrophenone

Domperidone is an antagonist of dopamine receptors, but acts mainly at peripheral sites as it does not readily cross the blood-brain barrier. As such it will have direct actions on gastric motility and a lower incidence of extrapyramidal effects than other dopamine receptor antagonists like the phenothiazines and metoclopramide.

The standard dose (20 mg orally qds or six hourly) is effective in 50–60% of patients receiving non-cisplatin chemotherapy (D'Souza et al., 1980) and is also effective against radiotherapy-induced nausea and vomiting (Reyntjens, 1979).

Domperidone has a good side-effect profile and is suitable, therefore, in combination therapy. It is also welcome in paediatric oncology, since children are extremely sensitive to the extrapyramidal effects of metoclopramide.

In postoperative nausea and vomiting domperidone is superior to metoclopramide, but not as effective as droperidol (Korttila et al., 1979). Generally it appears to be more efficient in treating than preventing PONV (Palazzo & Strunin, 1984b).

The intravenous preparation of domperidone has been withdrawn in the UK following reports of cardiac dysrythmias after using this route of administration. This may limit its use in PONV since the intramuscular route of administration has been shown to be ineffective (Korttila et al., 1979).

Phenothiazines

Originally synthesized in the late 19th century by chemists in the dye industry, the phenothiazines were found in the 1930s to have hypnotic properties. Since the 1950s they have been most widely used as anti-emetics. However they display several toxicities which limit their use, including extrapyramidal reactions, autonomic responses, hypersensitivity and hormonal dysfunction (Wampler, 1983). Furthermore the EPR liability of these drugs is cumulative and outlasts their anti-emetic action (Clarke, 1984).

Prochlorperazine is well known for treating chemotherapy-induced nausea and vomiting but close inspection of clinical trials reveal that at conventional doses it only exceeds placebo in efficacy (Orr et al., 1980), and is not as effective as THC, nabilone, high-dose metoclopramide or dexamethasone (reviewed in Bakowski, 1984). It is not very effective against the more emetogenic drugs. A more recent study has suggested that higher doses may be more effective but there is undoubtedly a dose-related increase in toxicity, especially hypotension, extrapyramidal reactions and sedation (Olver et al., 1989).

Phenothiazines, particularly prochlorperazine is used in PONV. Prochlorperazine reduced nausea and vomiting in 40–70% of patients in three separate studies, when used prophylactically. However two other studies have not been able to demonstrate efficacy (Rowbotham, 1992). Good anti-emetic efficacy was shown when prochlorperazine was give to treat established vomiting after anaesthesia (Loeser et al., 1979).

Phenothiazines are also used in treating vertigo, Ménière's disease and migraine.

Other phenothiazines are trifluoperazine, thiethylperazine, perphenazine and chlorpromazine. Of the whole group, chlorpromazine is the most effective anti-emetic, but it does have the problem of causing EPRs and hypotension. Chlorpromazine is not very effective against cisplatin-induced chemotherapy and only controls vomiting in around 50% of patients who have vomiting due to non-cisplatin regimens (Cunningham et al., 1985b). Chlorpromazine can induce sleep in patients who are still recovering from surgery (Palazzo & Strunin, 1984b). Chlorpromazine has no effect on motion sickness but promethazine is useful in this indication.

Steroids

Dexamethasone and methylprednisolone are the usual synthetic glucocorticosteroids employed as anti-emetics in cancer chemotherapy. The pharmacological actions of corticosteroids that account for their anti-emetic activity are unclear although it has been suggested that they stabilize cell membranes and decrease permeability of the blood-brain barrier. It has also been proposed that they inhibit the cerebral oedema (and hence raised intracranial pressure) that can be caused by cytotoxic drugs and radiation (Young, 1986). Steroids are usually only encountered as anti-emetics in cancer treatment; they are not employed for PONV or other types of emesis.

Given as a single agent methylprednisolone is only moderately effective; controlling emesis in 54% of patients receiving a variety of chemotherapy regimens (Rich et al., 1980) or only 16% of patients receiving cisplatin (Benrubi et al., 1985). It is more widely used in the USA than in the UK.

Single agent dexamethasone is more effective; it can control emesis in around 83% of patients on non-cisplatin regimens (Cassileth et al., 1983), and 71% of patients receiving moderate doses of cisplatin (Aapro & Alberts, 1981). It is superior to placebo, prochloperazine and intermediate dose metoclopramide (McDermed, 1983; D'Olimpio et al., 1984).

Steroids may have an important role in delayed emesis after chemotherapy (see Chapter 2). Dexamethasone has been shown to be comparable to ondansetron in controlling the delayed emesis after moderately emetogenic chemotherapy (Jones *et al.*, 1991) and a combination of dexamethasone plus ondansetron has been demonstrated to be the most effective anti-emetic combination to date for the treatment of delayed emesis due to cisplatin (Italian Group for Antiemetic Research, 1992).

Corticosteroids, particularly dexamethasone have a wide application in combination with other anti-emetic compounds, especially metoclopramide and ondansetron (see section on combination anti-emetic therapy).

Dexamethasone must be injected slowly to avoid perineal itching or scrotal pain. Long-term use of systemic steroids is not desirable due to their well known effects on the immune system and the production of Cushing-like symptoms.

Benzodiazepines

Benzodiazepines are sedatives and anxiolytics. Diazepam and lorazepam are probably the most common. Lorazepam is used extensively in psychiatry but was reported to have anti-emetic activity in the early 1980s. Lorazepam is used widely for treating chemotherapy-induced nausea and vomiting but is rarely employed for other types of emesis.

As a single agent its anti-emetic activity is limited (Laszlo *et al.*, 1985) but it has amnesic and anxiolytic activity; this may help patients tolerate treatment and may be exploited in the treatment of anticipatory emesis. One study has shown that 40% of patients did not remember their treatment and 80% experienced no significant anxiety (Laszlo *et al.*, 1985). Another study has concluded that lorazepam aids post-therapy symptom experience by decreasing fatigue and pain (Simms *et al.*, 1993).

Drowsiness is experienced by almost all patients and this is the reason it is included in many combination regimens. However this sedation may preclude its use in an out-patient setting.

Cannabinoids

Cannabinoids are a group of compounds extracted from the Indian hemp plant, *Cannabis sativa* L. Perhaps better known as marijuana (hashish, grass, weed, pot), its curative and euphoric properties have long been exploited in some cultures where it is taken as an infusion or, more often, smoked.

The anti-emetic action of cannabinoids was noted in the 1960s and 1970s in the USA when patients who were regular users of marijuana were noted to have lower incidence of nausea and vomiting than would be expected after chemotherapy. The isolation of the active agent, delta-9-tetrahydrocannabinol (THC) allowed more controlled clinical trials to take place.

THC has proved superior to placebo and prochlorperazine for treatment of chemotherapy induced emesis (Sallan *et al.*, 1980). However, as might be predicted, optimal anti-emetic control is associated with varying degrees of CNS disturbance (up to 30% of patients) as well as hypotension and dizziness. Such CNS disturbances (euphoria, dysphoria, hallucinations) are found particularly unacceptable by elderly patients.

The action of cannabinoids as an anti-emetic and indeed as a hallucinogen are not understood. Some degree of anxiolytic activity may contribute to the anti-emetic properties. They may also have anti-opioid activity.

Nabilone is a semisynthetic cannabinoid structurally related to THC and one of the few compounds developed specifically to be an anti-emetic. It has better bioavailability than THC and less effect on the cardiovascular system. Given as a single agent it is equal or superior to prochlorperazine and haloperidol (Steele *et al.*, 1980). It produces a similar incidence of euphoria or dysphoria to THC, but the incidence of CNS side-effects can be reduced by co-administration of prochlorperazine (Cunningham *et al.*, 1985a).

As a lipid soluble drug, nabilone can accumulate after repeat doses. Nabilone is not very effective against cisplatin-induced emesis, although it may prove useful with carboplatin. (Cunningham *et al.*, 1988).

Cannabinoids do not seem to be used as anti-emetics in any other areas of medicine.

Substituted benzamides

Metoclopramide is probably one of the most widely used anti-emetics being employed extensively for radio- and chemo-therapy-induced emesis, PONV, upper gastrointestinal disturbances and in some preparations for relief of migraine. It is a substituted benzamide. At low doses it antagonizes dopamine receptors, but at higher doses it is a 5-HT$_3$ receptor antagonist. This pharmacology is reflected in its anti-emetic activity. At low doses although useful for non-ulcer dyspepsia, irritable bowel syndrome, oesophageal reflux and some mild forms of vomiting it is a poor anti-emetic against chemotherapy-induced symptoms. At high doses it is effective against both non-cisplatin and cisplatin-containing chemotherapy regimens.

Metoclopramide stimulates gastric motility and is used before unplanned surgery to increase gastric emptying and minimize the risks associated with vomiting during anaesthesia. Because of this activity metoclopramide should not be given to patients who have undergone gastrointestinal surgery.

When used initially in oncology it was employed at oral doses of 10 mg three times daily. In some studies this proved no better than placebo and less effective than domperidone or THC. The intermediate dose of 20 mg three times daily is also poorly anti-emetic. Metoclopramide was shown to be a far more successful anti-emetic when the dose was increased to 2 mg/kg (a total of around 140 mg in an average man) administered over 15 minutes every two to three hours for three to six doses. This controlled emesis in 40% of patients receiving cisplatin chemotherapy. (For review of all these studies see Gralla, 1983.)

Subsequent studies showed that efficacy could be improved even further by adopting continuous rather than intermittent infusion as the method of administration (Warrington *et al.*, 1986); 81% of patients had major control of emesis (complete control was not recorded). A continuous infusion allows a steady plasma level of drug to be established and prevents the wide fluctuations in plasma levels seen with intermittent dosing. This allowed attainment of a serum level of 850–1000 ng/ml – levels consistent with optimum control of emesis (Meyer *et al.*, 1984).

Until the late 1980s high dose metoclopramide was probably the most effective single agent anti-emetic for cancer patients, being superior to chlorpromazine, prochlorperazine, haloperidol, tetrahydrocannabinol or dexamethasone (for review see Gralla *et al.*, 1987). However high dose metoclopramide is not as effective as the 5-HT_3 receptor antagonists for treating emesis in both non-cisplatin and cisplatin-containing regimens (Schmoll, 1989; Marty, 1990).

Although widely used in surgery its efficacy is controversial; approximately 50% of studies have shown that it is no more effective than placebo (Rowbotham, 1992). It has shown poor activity when administered with the pre-medication and is effective as a prophylactic medication only when given at the end of surgery (Handley, 1967; Lind & Breivik, 1970). Despite trying various dosing schedules a consistent anti-emetic action of metoclopramide has not been demonstrated in postoperative patients (Tornetta, 1969; Ellis & Spence, 1970; Shah & Wilson, 1972; Assaf *et al.*, 1974).

In cancer patients the most common side-effects of metoclopramide are sedation (60%), diarrhoea (15-30%) and EPRs which may develop in up to 20% of patients (Cunningham *et al.*, 1988). These EPRs are inevitably more common with higher doses of metoclopramide and are more prevalent in patients under 30 years of age. They are particularly common in children, up to 50% of whom may be affected. If occurring EPRs may be treated by procyclidine, intravenous benzhexol (2 mg), benztropine (2 mg) or, less commonly, diazepam (5–10 mg). It is contra-indicated after abdominal surgery.

5-HT₃ receptor antagonists

The 5-HT$_3$ receptor antagonists are the latest anti-emetic drugs to be developed. They were synthesized specifically as anti-emetics on the basis of experimental evidence (see sections 2.12 and 2.13) and were first introduced as anti-emetics for radio- and chemotherapy-induced nausea and vomiting. The first 5-HT$_3$ receptor antagonist available was ondansetron, followed by granisetron and tropisetron, although others are in development.

As a single agent 5-HT$_3$ receptor antagonists are the most effective anti-emetics we have for controlling radiotherapy and chemotherapy-induced emesis. The superior activity of ondansetron compared with high dose metoclopramide in cisplatin-induced emesis has been demonstrated (De Mulder *et al.*, 1990; Marty *et al.*, 1990; Hainsworth *et al.*, 1991).

Granisetron is as effective as the combination therapy of metoclopramide with dexamethasone (Chevallier, 1990) and tropisetron is superior to metoclopramide plus lorazepam (Dogliotti *et al.*, 1992).

In non-cisplatin-induced emesis very high levels of control of emesis, superior to any comparator anti-emetic, have been shown using ondansetron (Schmoll *et al.*, 1989; Marschner *et al.*, 1991), granisetron (Marty, 1990; Smith, 1990) and tropisetron (Bruijn, 1992).

In radiotherapy ondansetron is superior to metoclopramide in patients receiving high dose radiotherapy to the upper abdomen (Priestman *et al.*, 1990) and effective in patients receiving total body irradiation (TBI) in preparation for bone marrow transplantation (Schwella *et al.*, 1994). Tropisetron has been shown to be effective in women undergoing radiotherapy for ovarian cancer (Sorbe & Berglind, 1992) and granisetron is effective in patients undergoing lower hemibody irradiation (Logue *et al.*, 1991; Prentice, 1992).

Recent studies have shown that the clinical profile of the 5-

HT$_3$ receptor antagonists are similar in terms of efficacy and side effects for the control of acute nausea and vomiting.

In non-cisplatin-induced chemotherapy ondansetron and granisetron gave similar results for control of acute nausea and vomiting and patient preference was equally divided between the two (Bonneterre & Hecquet, 1993). Ondansetron and granisetron gave similar control rates of emesis over five days of fractionated chemotherapy (Dilly, 1993).

In acute cisplatin-induced emesis control of nausea and vomiting, patient preference and side effects were not statistically different for ondansetron and granisetron (Ruff *et al.*, 1994).

One study has looked at the control of acute emesis by all three drugs in moderately emetogenic chemotherapy. No overall superiority could be ascribed to any one 5-HT$_3$ receptor antagonist, although fewer treatment failures occurred with granisetron (Jantunen *et al.*, 1993). This study must be interpreted with caution, since there is no indication as to whether the data were analysed for interaction between treatment and course number or treatment differences. Emetic responses to chemotherapy are known to change over different cycles of treatment.

Many cancer nurses regard 5-HT$_3$ receptor antagonists as having had a major impact on chemotherapy-induced nausea and vomiting and feel that it is now possible to offer patients a degree of symptom control that was not previously easy to obtain. There is no doubt that 5-HT$_3$ receptor antagonists have proved useful in patients who previously responded poorly to more conventional anti-emetics (Bruntsch *et al.*, 1992; Blieberg *et al.*, 1992).

The 5-HT$_3$ receptor antagonists are also recommended for delayed emesis. However the marked superiority of 5-HT$_3$ receptor antagonists over other anit-emetics is not maintained for delayed emesis (De Mulder *et al.*, 1990; Jones *et al.*, 1991; Marty 1990; Chevallier *et al.*, 1990; Venner, 1990). The situation is not the same when combination anti-emetics are used (see below).

In view of the incidence of EPRs in children and younger adults (<30 years) with dopamine receptor antagonists the 5-HT$_3$ receptor antagonists are particularly useful in this group of patients. Ondansetron is the only 5-HT$_3$ receptor antagonist specifically licensed for paediatric use and has been shown to be safe and effective in children (Pinkerton *et al.*, 1990).

All 5-HT$_3$ receptor antagonists have a similar side effect profile in that they cause mild constipation and headache in around 5% and 10% of patients respectively. Importantly, they do not act on dopamine receptors and are, therefore, not likely to cause extrapyramidal reactions.

One 5-HT$_3$ receptor antagonist, ondansetron, has been licensed for use in PONV. Ondansetron has been shown to be effective in both prevention and treatment of PONV (Russell & Kenny, 1992; Dupeyron *et al.*, 1993). It has no effect on time to recover from anaesthetic (Lessin *et al.*, 1991) and does not cause respiratory depression (Frazer *et al.*, 1991) so it is suitable for both in-patient and out-patient use.

Combination anti-emetic therapy

The nausea and vomiting induced by cancer chemotherapy, especially cisplatin-containing chemotherapy, has historically been difficult to control. For this reason most cancer units adopt a process of using a combination or 'cocktail' of anti-emetic drugs. The basis of this approach is to combine anti-emetics with different modes of action to enhance overall anti-emetic control.

This has advantages of being able to treat different causes of emesis simultaneously. For example lorazepam may decrease a patient's anxiety while a 5-HT$_3$ receptor antagonist will control the action of 5-HT released by chemotherapy.

Steroids are particularly useful in combination therapy as they have been shown to increase the efficacy of metoclopramide (Allan *et al.*, 1984) and ondansetron (Roila *et al.*, 1990; Smyth *et al.*, 1991) and other drugs such as domperidone.

Care must be taken to ensure that the side-effect profile of combination anti-emetics remains acceptable. Sometimes the role of one of the components of an anti-emetic cocktail is to reduce the side-effects induced by other drugs (iatrogenic side-effects). Thus the side-effects of metoclopramide can be reduced by the addition of lorazepam or diphenhydramine (Benrubi *et al.*, 1985; Kris *et al.*, 1987; Roila *et al.*, 1989). Procyclidine is also used to reduce the risks of EPRs. Counteracting side effects is not always the best course of action and it may be more acceptable to select a drug with a better side-effect profile in the first place.

The most commonly used anti-emetic 'cocktails' are domperidone plus lorazepam, domperidone plus dexamethasone, chlorpromazine plus dexamethasone or nabilone plus prochlorperazine and metoclopramide plus dexamethasone plus diphenhydramine or lorazepam. Ondansetron and granisetron are given with dexamethasone where high levels of anti-emetic control are required. Most oncology units would now give a 5-HT_3 receptor antagonist plus dexamethasone to patients receiving the most highly emetogenic chemotherapy, as it is simpler regimen and has fewer side-effects than other combinations.

One study has shown that patients who received ondansetron plus dexamethasone continued with better anti-emetic control during the delayed emesis period than those who received a combination of metoclopramide, dexamethasone and diphenhydramine even though both groups were given the same anti-emetic regimen (metoclopramide plus dexamethasone) for the delayed emesis period (Italian Group for Antiemetic Research, 1992).

Choosing an appropriate anti-emetic

The choice of an appropriate anti-emetic will depend upon a variety of factors: the cause of the nausea and vomiting, patient demographic factors, in-patient or day case use, the appropriateness and acceptability of the drug formulation (tablet, injection), the risk of EPRs and the preferences or previous experience of the prescribing doctor or nurse.

It is not possible to give firm recommendations for suitable anti-emetics in each situation but Table 4.2 summarizes some of the important properties of the drugs to be considered.

When the nausea and vomiting is being caused by a drug, for example an antibiotic or antiviral compound, it is often easier to change the drug to one that does not cause emesis or to take care in how the drug is given. For example dividing doses or giving the drug with food will often circumvent the problem.

The nausea and vomiting caused by SSRI anti-depressant drugs is likely to respond well to 5-HT_3 receptor antagonists as the emesis they induce is due to raised 5-HT levels. However this has yet to be evaluated in the clinical setting.

The anti-Parkinsonian drugs cause nausea and vomiting by raising central dopamine levels. Giving an anti-dopaminergic anti-emetic would therefore be defeating the object of the main drug. There is evidence that the emesis caused by L-dopa, the main treatment for Parkinsonism, is peripheral in origin since carbidopa which is given with L-dopa can attenuate L-dopa-induced emesis in animals (Liotti & Clark, 1974). Carbidopa prevents peripheral decarboxylation of L-dopa to dopamine but being unable to cross the blood-brain barrier does not affect central dopamine. A suitable anti-emetic in these circumstances might therefore be domperidone which does not cross the blood-brain barrier readily.

Table 4.2 Summary of anti-emetic uses

Class of anti-emetic	Uses	Side-effects	Special notes
anticholinergic	motion sickness, PONV	Drowsiness, dizziness, visual disturbances, dry mouth	'Central cholinergic syndrome' can occur in the elderly Hyoscine patches are useful for travel sickness
antihistamines	motion sickness, vertigo, labyrinthine disorders, chemotherapy, radiotherapy	Drowsiness, sedation	Component of many OTC preparations for motion sickness For highly emetogenic chemotherapy only Useful as part of an anti-emetic 'cocktail'
butyrophenones	PONV, chemotherapy	Sedation, EPRs, mild hypotension	
substituted butyrophenone	PONV, chemotherapy, L-dopa-induced, gastrointestinal disturbances	Less EPRs than other dopamine receptor antagonists as it does not cross the blood-brain barrier readily	
phenothiazines	PONV, chemotherapy, radiotherapy, vertigo, migraine	EPRs, dry mouth, hypotension	Most common anti-emetic group for PONV
corticosteroids	chemotherapy, radiotherapy	For short-term use side-effects are minor. Long-term use can cause Cushingoid symptoms and depression of the immune system	Widely used in 'cocktails'. Recommended for delayed emesis Must be injected slowly to avoid perineal itching and burning or scrotal pain
benzodiazepines	PONV, chemotherapy, radiotherapy	Drowiness, confusion respiratory depression at high doses	Amnesic properties can help in ANV. Useful given the night before treatment
cannabinoids	chemotherapy	Can cause euphoria, hallucinations, dysphoria	Unsuitable for elderly patients
substituted benzamides	chemotherapy, radiotherapy, IBS, non-ulcer dyspepsia, gastrointestinal disorders, PONV	EPRs – especially in children, diarrhoea, sedation	High doses needed for cisplatin chemotherapy can cause EPRs. Contra-indicated after gastric surgery. Used to promote gastric emptying before emergency surgery
5-HT₃ receptor antagonists	chemotherapy, radiotherapy, PONV	Headache, constipation	Only ondansetron is available for PONV

Where nausea is the predominant problem without vomiting and especially if there is identifiable gastric stasis then a prokinetic, such as cisapride, may be most useful.

Selection of anti-emetics is particularly difficult in chemotherapy clinics since there are a variety of chemotherapy regimens with different emetic potentials, and patient factors will influence how different individuals can respond to the same chemotherapy drugs. Table 4.3 suggests some possible anti-emetic regimens, but again this should not be taken as a firm recommendation.

Anti-emetics for terminally ill patients

For obvious reasons comparative trials of anti-emetic drugs are rarely (if ever) carried out in terminally ill patients. Experience in the palliative care setting has however accumulated valuable empirical experience which demonstrates the usefulness of several anti-emetic agents.

When patients are suffering from bowel obstruction or the cause of the nausea and vomiting are unknown then cyclizine plus haloperidol or hyoscine plus haloperidol have proved useful. Cyclizine is given four hourly and haloperidol 12 hourly or the two drugs can be combined and can be given subcutaneously over 24 hours through a syringe driver (Finlay, 1991). Hyoscine can be given orally every eight hours, subcutaneously over 24 hours or transdermally for three days (Regnard & Comiskey, 1992). The 5-HT$_3$ receptor antagonist ondansetron has also been suggested for these conditions (Regnard & Comiskey, 1992).

These regimens have proved particularly useful in cases of subacute obstruction and have circumvented the need for hospitalization during the latter stages of the disease. Drugs which stimulate motility, such as metoclopramide, should be avoided in cases of obstruction where they can increase discomfort.

More recently the strategy of relieving the symptoms of gastrointestinal obstruction by reducing the volume of gastric contents has been investigated. Orectide, a somatostatin analogue, reduces intestinal fluid secretion and improves electrolyte absorption. This drug has been used successfully as a subcutaneous injection in terminally ill patients with bowel obstruction; its use controlling vomiting, decreasing the need for anti-emetics (Mercadante *et al.*, 1993).

Corticosteroids have an anti-emetic action in chemotherapy-induced emesis. Their activity in reducing tissue oedema may provide an added benefit where tumour bulk is a problem.

Table 4.3 Summary of suitable anti-emetics for use with chemotherapy

Emetic potential – classified as in Table 3.3	Anti-emetics for acute emesis	Anti-emetics for delayed emesis
<10%	Lorazepam	
Class I (<10%)	Lorazepam 1–2 mg po bd/tds OR domperidone 20 mg po qds	
Class II (10–30%)	prochlorperazine 12.5–25 mg iv 3–6 hourly/ 5–10 mg po 4–6 hourly OR dexamethasone 8 mg with chemo. then OR metoclopramide 10–20 mg tds	dexamethasone 4 mg po tds for 3 days
Class III (30–60%)	metoclopramide 30–100 mg iv + dexamethasone 4–8 mg iv OR dexamethasone 8 mg iv stat OR domperidone supp 30 mg 6 hourly + lorazepam 1–2 mg iv OR ondansetron 8 mg po bd OR granisetron 1 mg po OR tropisetron 5 mg iv/po	dexamethasone 4 mg tds po for 2 days + metoclopramide 20 mg qds for 3 days ondansetron 8 mg po bd up to 5 days tropisetron 5 mg po up to 5 days
Class IV (60–90%)	ondansetron 8–32 mg iv before chemo OR granisetron 3 mg iv before chemo OR tropisetron 5 mg iv before chemo OR metoclopramide 2 mg/kg 2–4 hourly + dexamethasone 8 mg iv + lorazepam 1–2 mg	ondansetron 8 mg po bd up to 5 days OR dexamethasone 4 mg tds po 2 days + metoclopramide 20 mg qds for 3 days
Class V (>90%)	ondansetron 8–32 mg + dexamethasone 8–20 mg	ondansetron 8 mg po bd for up to 5 days OR metoclopramide 20 mg qds + dexamethasone 4 mg tds po

These doses are taken from the literature; they are guidelines only and the manufacturer's data sheet should be consulted for full information.

Reduction in tumour mass can alleviate obstruction or localized pressure e.g. from brain metastases.

Haloperidol is also used for opiate-induced nausea and vomiting in terminal patients, although the reason why it should be effective is not immediately obvious. Domperidone has proved useful where hepatic metastases or constipation are the main causes of the nausea and vomiting. If excessive bronchial secretions are a contributory factor to patient discomfort hyoscine has proved useful (Finlay, 1991).

Timing of anti-emetic administration

It is a general rule that it is easier to prevent emesis from occurring than to stop it once it has started. So in situations where vomiting is a predictable side-effect, such as after cancer treatment or postoperatively it is best to give anti-emetics prophylactically. Avoiding vomiting from the outset is also preferable for patient comfort.

The anti-emetic must also be given time to take effect. If it is to be given by injection it will probably be effective almost immediately, but tablets or suppositories need time to be absorbed. A tablet is also of little use to someone who is actively vomiting. Where anxiolytics are being used they are best given several hours before treatment, often the night before.

In the surgical setting it may be easy to 'top-up' a dose of anti-emetic during surgery via a cannula that is in place but after surgery the patient may wish to avoid injections. Tablets are often not appropriate postoperatively if normal gastrointestinal function has not resumed.

It is important, therefore, to use the dosages and routes of administration recommended as these have been devised making use of the pharmacokinetic properties of the anti-emetic. More information on administration of anti-emetics is given in Chapter 6.

Summary of Chapter 4

- Anti-emetic drugs comprise a variety of different types of drugs, many of which are pharmacologically complex.
- Most anti-emetics have some side-effects, the main undesirable side-effects being sedation and extra-pyramidal reactions (EPRs). Young patients and those receiving anti-emetics on consecutive days are particularly prone to EPRs.

- Recently a new class of anti-emetic compounds – the 5-HT_3 receptor antagonists – have been developed specifically to treat emesis. These agents are proving superior to other single agent anti-emetics and are not likely to cause EPRs or sedation.
- 5-HT_3 receptor antagonist are effective in radiotherapy and chemotherapy-induced nausea and vomiting and one 5-HT_3 receptor antagonist, ondansetron, is also used in PONV.
- A summary of the commonly prescribed anti-emetics and the combination regimens used most widely in chemotherapy are given.

SELF ASSESSMENT QUESTIONS

1. Extrapyramidal reactions (EPRs):

                                                           TRUE   FALSE

   (a) are more common in children

   (b) are due to antagonism of serotonin receptors

   (c) often start with feelings of a swollen tongue

   (d) include sedation

   (e) are seen in Parkinson's disease

   (f) cannot be treated

2. The improved efficacy of metoclopramide at high doses is due to its action on:

   (a) central D_2 receptors

   (b) both central and peripheral D_2 receptors

   (c) peripheral and central $5\text{-}HT_3$ receptors

   (d) central H_2 receptors

3. Sedation is a side-effect of:

   (a) prochlorperazine

   (b) ondansetron

   (c) high-dose metoclopramide

   (d) lorazepam

   (e) haloperidol

4. Match the drugs on the left with one or more side effects on the right:

A. metodopramide	1. confusion	A
B. prochlorperazine	2. dysphoria	B
C. THC	3. constipation	C
D. ondansetron	4. hypotension	D
	5. dry mouth	
	6. EPRs	

5. Are the following statements true
   or false?   TRUE   FALSE

   (a) ondansetron is superior to high-dose
       metoclopramide for cisplatin-
       induced vomiting
   (b) lorazepam has amnesic properties
   (c) 5-HT$_3$ receptor antagonists are the
       only group of drugs developed
       specifically for treating emesis
   (d) intravenous domperidone is not
       recommended

6. Indicate with a tick which drugs have
   proven efficacy in PONV:

   (a) metoclopramide
   (b) prochlorperazine
   (c) nabilone
   (d) dexamethasone
   (e) ondansetron

7. The 5-HT$_3$ receptor antagonists: TRUE   FALSE

   (a) are unlikely to cause EPRs
   (b) can be administered by continuous
       intravenous infusion
   (c) are not effective in radiation induced
       emesis

8. Benzodiazepines:

   (a) are useful in treating anticipatory
       nausea and vomiting
   (b) have useful amnesic effects
   (c) can be administered in high doses
       intravenously to out-patients
   (d) may cause respiratory depression

9. Cannabinoids: TRUE   FALSE

   (a) are particularly useful in children
   (b) can be administered two hourly if
       required
   (c) can cause hallucinations or
       dysphoria

10. Are the following statements true or
    false?

    (a) dexamethasone is best given as a
        rapid bolus injection
    (b) anti-emetics should be given before
        chemo- or radiotherapy
    (c) prochlorperazine and
        chlorpromazine are useful in
        suppository form
    (d) sedatives should be avoided the night
        before treatment

11. Combination anti-emetic therapies:

    (a) are more effective than single agent
        regimens
    (b) cannot mix oral and intravenous
        drugs
    (c) never include prochloperazine
    (d) often utilize dexamethasone

12. Which of the following drugs would be
    best suited for use in combination with
    metoclopramide?

    (a) dexamethasone
    (b) nabilone
    (c) ondansetron
    (d) haloperidol

13. Lorazepam is used in combination
    therapy because: TRUE   FALSE

    (a) it has amnesic properties
    (b) it causes sedation
    (c) it increases the gastrointestinal
        activity
    (d) it can reduce anxiety

14. Are the following true or false?

    (a) dopamine receptor antagonists are
        most useful in children
    (b) out-patients appreciate sedating anti-
        emetics
    (c) dexamethasone should be injected
        rapidly
    (d) anti-emetics should be given after
        chemotherapy

15. In cases of gastrointestinal obstruction in
    terminally ill patients:

    (a) metoclopramide should be avoided
    (b) orectide has proved useful
    (c) cyclizine should not be given
    (d) 5-HT$_3$ receptor antagonists are not
        useful

CHAPTER 5: NATURAL PRODUCTS AND SUPPORTIVE TECHNIQUES FOR EMESIS CONTROL

Techniques that are not part of conventional medicine are know by a variety of names: alternative, complementary, supportive. In this book supportive techniques is the preferred term.

The last two decades have seen a narrowing of the gulf between supportive techniques and conventional medicine. People have become more open to the suggestions of using supportive techniques, sometimes alongside or as an adjunct to prescription medicines. More and more health care professionals are abandoning their initial scepticism and accepting that even if supportive techniques are unsuitable regimens for controlling or curing disease, they can have a place in controlling side-effects, in raising patients' morale and improving their sense of well-being.

This chapter considers how some naturally occurring compounds and supportive techniques can help patients cope with nausea and vomiting. Perhaps it is not surprising that by far the greatest interest in supportive techniques is in the area of cancer care. It is really only in the longer-term treatment situation that techniques such as relaxation, hypnosis, guided imagery can be given sufficient time to be effective. Less time consuming techniques, such as acupressure or acupuncture, are used in surgical patients or pregnant women.

5.1 Natural products for controlling emesis

In animal experiments emesis induced by cisplatin has been controlled by feverfew (Rudd & Naylor, 1990) and the ginger extract 6-gingerol (Yamahara *et al.*, 1989a). Both of these actions may be related to 5-HT since feverfew can release 5-HT from platelets and 6-gingerol is active in a system used for assaying the 5-HT$_3$ receptor – although how selective this action was is not known (Yamahara *et al.*, 1989b). Ginger root has also been shown to be more effective than placebo in controlling PONV (Bone *et al.*, 1990).

These results do not provide sufficient evidence to suggest that natural products could replace effective pharmaceutical preparations. For patients in whom the nausea and vomiting is severe, such as cancer patients, nurses should adhere to any prescribed schedule of medication.

However in less clinically serious situations there may be a place for natural remedies. There is a tendency to assume that if a product is 'natural' it must therefore be safe. This is not always true (there are many naturally poisonous plants) and it must be remembered that naturally occurring products do have pharmacological actions and the normal caution of not giving any drugs to pregnant women should be observed.

5.2 Relief of anxiety

Anxiety is a factor that contributes to the amount of emesis which occurs (see Chapter 3). Many supportive techniques are aimed at reducing or relieving anxiety and producing a calming influence on the patient. This may be achieved to a certain extent by the nurse's approach; a calm and positive attitude and a few well chosen words can do much to relieve anxiety. For maximum benefit more overt behaviourial interventions are required.

The most commonly used techniques are relaxation, progressive muscle relaxation therapy/training (PMRT), hypnosis, guided imagery, systematic desensitization and acupuncture or acupressure.

The basis of the majority of these techniques is relaxation. The techniques differ only in the way that relaxation is induced. Guided imagery is used in conjunction with relaxation, PMRT, hypnosis or systematic desensitization. It too is a form of relaxing the patient.

5.3 Relaxation

Nurses and doctors frequently use phrases like 'relax and this won't be so bad' under circumstances ranging from giving injections, inserting a catheter, removing stitches or just taking off a plaster. Relaxation is the extension of this phrase into a whole technique that enables the patient to do just that. Relaxation techniques may be practised on an individual basis or patients can be taught in groups or classes. It is often nurses or physiotherapists who run such groups but other health care professionals (e.g. psychologists) may be involved.

The therapist must aim to create a non-threatening, undisturbed and friendly environment. The patient must be made comfortable and attention paid to surroundings – lighting and temperature must be appropriate and soothing music or gentle background sounds, such as sea-sounds, are often played. The therapist then takes the patient(s) through a routine that induces relaxation. Usually routines pass through several stages each of which promotes deeper relaxation. The techniques involve a commentary which generally suggests warmth, comfort, heaviness, etc.

A teaching plan for teaching relaxation therapy to cancer patients is given by Copley Cobb (1984).

5.4 Progressive muscle relaxation therapy

Alternatively, PMRT is employed where the patient is taught to become aware of the tension in each part of the body, to contract and tense muscles and then 'let go' and relax completely. The process of tensing and relaxing is carried out in a step-by-step fashion, usually moving from feet to head. PMRT is not suitable for weak or debilitated patients in whom the physical exertion required may be unsuitable.

5.5 Guided imagery

Guided imagery is a particular type of relaxation procedure. During the commentary to help relaxation, images are introduced which assist the process. The patient may be asked to imagine a soft, warm cloth wiping away the tension. Alternatively the patient may be asked to retrieve from memory a pleasing visual image. The image is frequently a person or place associated with pleasurable memories or satisfaction. The therapist might suggest a scene that will appeal to most people – a sandy beach, warm blue sea, a spring meadow or a lovely hot bath. Patients are asked to examine this image in some detail, to visualize the colours, hear the sounds involved, feel the air on their skin, notice the temperature, feel the sunshine on their bodies and so on. Once explored in such detail this image can then easily be recalled to assist in relaxation. Therapists will develop their own routine. A complete script of relaxation with guided imagery is given in Donovan (1980).

Patients vary in the amount of training they require. Some

may take four or five practice sessions before they note any effects; others appreciate changes immediately.

It is apparent that part of these techniques rely on distracting the patient from the immediate surroundings. Attentional diversion has indeed been a useful technique in relieving stress and pain (McCaul & Malott, 1984). It is likely that this aspect of relaxation training contributes to its efficacy in treating radio- and chemotherapy-induced nausea and vomiting.

5.6 Physiological changes associated with relaxation

Active relaxation techniques, as opposed to just being told 'sit and relax', have been shown to produce physiological responses in subjects under laboratory conditions. These responses include lowering of heart and respiration rates, decreases in muscle tension and decreases in skin conductance (see Cotanch, 1983). Similarly transcendental meditation has been shown to reduce oxygen consumption, cause a slowing in brain waves and reduce heart and respiration rates.

Relaxation training has been shown to have similar effects in cancer patients, although the sample number was quite small (Cotanch, 1983). Relaxation with guided imagery has also been shown to be effective in reducing nausea (Figure 5.1) and to have significant effects on blood pressure, heart rate and anxiety over four to five cycles of chemotherapy (Burish *et al.*, 1987). In both these studies patients were also receiving conventional anti-emetic drugs.

5.7 Therapeutic touch, massage and aromatherapy

'Whether we are young or old, the touch of another person is essential to our well-being, and never more so than when we are distressed and unwell' (Turton, 1989). This is undoubtedly true, and the concerned touch of another person can reduce stress and anxiety (Barnett, 1972), goals which are important in treating nausea and vomiting in patients.

However, the amount of touching people find acceptable in everyday life varies enormously with different cultures and the individual's own preferences. Casual touching is often not acceptable; for some people it may make them positively uncomfortable. Placing physical contact on a more formal

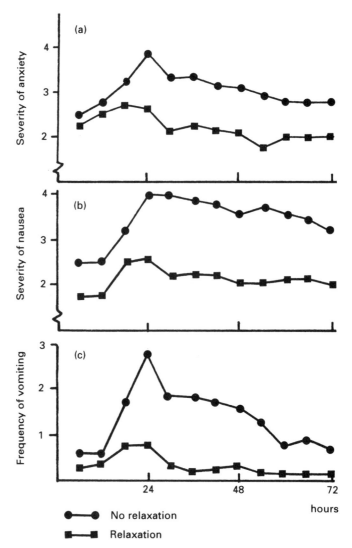

Figure 5.1 Effects of relaxation. Mean patient ratings of anxiety (a) nausea (b) and vomiting (c) in the 72 hours after chemotherapy. (Taken from Burish *et al.*, 1987. © 1987 American Psychological Association. Reprinted with permission.)

footing, where the process has a structure and the participants have well-defined roles, can make it more acceptable to some patients. This is not to suggest that contact should be forced on patients but where a patient is finding difficulty in communicating, physical contact with a nurse can often help in establishing relationships without offence or invasion of personal space (Byass, 1988).

In a hospice setting it was found that 'Through gentle massage with oils and herbs ... patients tend to open up and say what they are feeling and what their fears are. This, in turn, has enabled us to counsel more easily and deal with psychological pain as well as social and physical pain' (Tisserand, 1988).

Touching can, therefore, reduce anxiety and open up lines of communication. The techniques generally used in nursing are therapeutic touch, massage and aromatherapy.

Therapeutic touch can be defined as: the simple placing of the hands for about 10–15 minutes on, or close to, the body of an ill person by someone who intends to help or heal that person (Krieger, 1975). It has been shown that such techniques are valuable in pain relief (Boguslawski, 1980), but its role in anti-emesis has yet to be established.

Massage is manipulation of the soft tissues using four basic hand movements – stroking, kneading, percussion and friction. Such actions are thought to reduce muscle tension, improve circulation and lymph drainage, lower heart rate and blood pressure, increase trunk and limb flexibility and raise body and skin temperature (Turton, 1989).

Aromatherapy utilizes plant extracts, usually in the form of oils, to enhance the massages. Different plants are thought to have properties that help alleviate specific problems, such as headache, tension or insomnia.

While these techniques can be learned quite easily, some training by qualified personnel is usually required before an individual is able to employ these techniques. Massage should only be given by someone who has received formal training.

5.8 Comparative studies with anti-emetic drugs

Few studies have evaluated critically the anti-emetic efficacy of any supportive techniques and those studies which have been done are usually on a very small patient sample making it difficult to apply their results to the wider population.

One study gave relaxation therapy along with standard anti-emetics to 43 cancer patients and compared their responses with those of 24 matched controls who only received anti-emetics. There was no difference between the two groups (Holli, 1993).

A direct comparison has been made between relaxation with slow back massage and a standard anti-emetic drug regimen (Scott *et al.*, 1986). Patients with ovarian cancer who were to receive high-dose cisplatin plus doxorubicin and cyclophosphamide were allocated to relaxation therapy or anti-emetic drug therapy (combination of metoclopramide (2 mg/kg), dexamethasone (20 mg) and diphenhydramine (50 mg)).

The group receiving anti-emetic drugs had significantly less episodes of vomiting and the episodes were less intense. On average the group using relaxation had three times as many total emetic episodes as those in the drug group. However, the patients using relaxation techniques vomited for a shorter period (12 hours) than the drug group (17 hours).

This study should not be taken as evidence that relaxation does not work, for most practitioners would say the time devoted to relaxation training (one hour the night before plus a tape and opportunity to practise that evening) would be insufficient for most techniques. However these results and those presented above, where relaxation in combination with drugs proved superior to drugs alone, suggests that the role of relaxation may be in addition to rather than instead of conventional anti-emetic drugs.

This conclusion is reinforced by the study of Troesch and colleagues (1993) in patients receiving cisplatin chemotherapy. They showed that while the amount of nausea and vomiting was not reduced by using guided imagery the patients receiving supportive interventions expressed a more positive attitude, feeling more unafraid, in control, hopeful, powerful and relaxed than the non-guided imagery group.

Relaxation may, therefore, contribute to overall patient well-being.

5.9 Acupuncture or acupressure

Of all the supportive techniques available acupuncture and acupressure have probably been most thoroughly investigated.

Acupuncture is the ancient Chinese technique of stimulating well-defined points on the body to produce control of pain, relief from symptoms or cure of disease. The areas of the body lie on meridians which link internal organs with accessible cutaneous areas. Maps of such meridians have been in existence for hundreds of years – they are the acupuncturist's textbook of anatomy. Acupuncture involves inserting needles into these specific acupuncture points. The needles may then be rotated, heated or have a small electric current passed through them. Transcutaneous electrical stimuli can also be applied directly to the acupuncture point.

Acupressure is non-invasive and involves applying pressure to the acupuncture point.

The relevant point for the control of emesis is the P6 or the

Neiguan or Neikuan point, which lies on the pericardial meridian and is located on the inner surface of the wrist, three fingers width above the distal skin crease of the wrist joint between the tendons of *palmaris longus* and *flexor carpi radialis* (see Figure 5.2).

5.10 Advantages of acupressure

Acupressure is easier to administer than acupuncture and can be used safely on an out-patient basis. As it is non-invasive it is more acceptable to some patients. Furthermore acupuncture has been reported to be effective for approximately eight hours when used for anti-emesis which limits its usefulness. Although the acupuncture can be repeated during the risk period following chemotherapy, this is time consuming for the therapist and expensive for the oncology unit. Acupressure, on the other hand, can be used continuously by patients themselves.

Since publicity has been given to the anti-emetic action of acupressure, special wrist bands have become commercially available for this use. These are elasticated wrist bands that incorporate a small plastic stud which can be located over the P6 point (Figure 5.2). Known as 'Sea-bands'^{TM} or 'Travel-bands'^{TM} they have been marketed for treating sea-sickness and the 'morning sickness' of pregnancy as well as being used in cancer therapy. These products can reduce the cost of therapy as

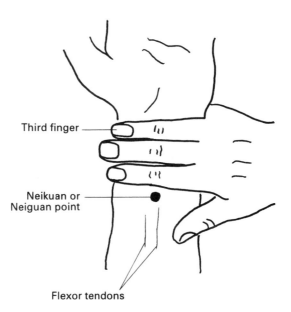

Figure 5.2 The Neikuan point. The wrist band is positioned on the Neikuan (or Neiguan) point for acupressure treatment of nausea and vomiting.

Third finger

Neikuan or Neiguan point

Flexor tendons

the only expenses involved are the initial cost of providing bands and instructing the patient in their use.

5.11 Procedure for using wrist bands

Usually a 'Sea-band'™ is placed upon each wrist immediately after chemotherapy has been administered. Some studies have used only the right wrist, as is the practice of conventional Chinese medicine, but there are indications that this may not be so effective, especially in left-handed patients. While a prophylactic approach is taken with most anti-emetic techniques, the sheer difficulty of administering chemotherapy via an intravenous line with a wrist band in position usually makes this impractical. Thus wrist bands are placed in position as soon as the administration of chemotherapy is completed. Patients are instructed to press the stud on the band at regular time intervals, recommendations vary but it is usually suggested that the patient presses the stud for two to five minutes every two or six hours.

5.12 Clinical studies

Clinical trials have shown that acupuncture and acupressure produce benefit in the majority of patients although the numbers involved are, as yet, small.

In a study of 105 patients who had troublesome sickness during a previous course of cisplatin chemotherapy (despite the use of anti-emetic drugs) 99 benefited from acupuncture (Dundee *et al.*, 1989) with 63% reporting complete relief of symptoms.

A further study gave an initial electrical stimulation of the P6 point followed by the use of wrist bands for the subsequent 24 hours. During this time the patients pressed the stud for five minutes every two hours. All the hospitalized and the majority (75%) of the out-patients studied received benefit from the acupressure (Dundee & Yang, 1990). Of the hospitalized patients, 80% had no sickness at all.

Acupressure alone has been shown to have significant effect in reducing postoperative nausea and the incidence of post-operative vomiting. The need for further anti-emetics was also reduced (Barsoum *et al.*, 1990).

Acupressure has been shown to produce significant ($p < 0.01$) and positive benefit in pregnant women, although a control group pressing a 'dummy' point instead of the real acupressure point also improved (p<0.05) (Dundee, 1988). This might be due to a significant psychological component of acupressure, however, the number of patients with no sickness was higher in the true acupressure group.

5.13 Psychological aspects of acupuncture

Traditional Chinese medical techniques are only poorly understood in the West. The controversy as to whether the benefit from acupuncture/acupressure is due to the patient's belief in the technique or whether there is a direct physiological action of stimulating the acupuncture point has raged for many years. It is unlikely to be resolved in the near future and such considerations are beyond the scope of this book. However the following points are worthy of consideration:

- Anecdotally it has been noted that the more anxious patients seem to benefit more from acupuncture/acupressure than those who are more calm and relaxed when they receive their chemotherapy.
- Pressing the acupressure stud gives patients an active involvement with their own treatment. It is quite disconcerting and bewildering for some patients to undergo therapy. They feel 'taken over' by the oncology team, no longer in control of their own body or life. Active involvement in the therapy restores some of the responsibility to the patient.
- Acupuncture given while a patient is anaesthetized and unaware of its administration, is less effective than acupuncture given before the pre-medication (Weightman *et al.*, 1987). This may be related to the timing of the acupuncture relative to the emetic stimulus (before or after opioid pre-medication) or to the awareness of the patient.
- Pregnant women who were shown a 'dummy' acupressure point near the elbow, also benefited from the procedure, although not to the same extent as the true acupressure group (Dundee, 1988).

It is likely, therefore, that a psychological component plays a part in the effectiveness of acupuncture.

5.14 Selecting patients for supportive therapy

It would appear that most supportive therapies used to control emesis are most useful as an adjunct rather than a replacement for conventional drug therapy. This is not to underestimate their value. For the patient in whom conventional drugs are not totally effective or where the distress of emesis is causing severe problems of loss of morale or anorexia, supportive techniques can be very valuable. Such systems cannot be used, however, with a patient who is unwilling or unco-operative. The commitment to the therapy must come from both nursing staff and patient. Although the psychological component can be disputed there is no doubt that such interventions have only limited success with patients who are cynical, sceptical or suspicious. Possible benefits must be measured against the time consuming commitment such programmes of treatment demand – from the patient and the nurse.

Summary of Chapter 5

- Supportive techniques are becoming more acceptable and widely used.
- Most supportive techniques aim at inducing relaxation and reducing anxiety.
- Acupuncture and acupressure have been investigated more than most other types of supportive therapy.
- Clinical trials, though limited, suggest that supportive techniques are best employed as an adjunct to rather than a substitute for anti-emetic drugs.
- Supportive techniques require time and commitment. Patients who will benefit must be selected with care.

SELF ASSESSMENT QUESTIONS

1. Rate as true or false:

   TRUE   FALSE

   (a) naturally occurring products are not pharmacologically active

   (b) ginger and feverfew have anti-emetic properties under experimental conditions

   (c) anxiety can be a contributory factor to all types of nausea and vomiting

2. Supportive anti-emetic techniques:

   (a) are only used in hospital

   (b) can improve the success of anti-emetic drugs

   (c) have less marked effects in anxious patients

   (d) do not help anticipatory nausea and vomiting

3. Relaxation techniques have been shown to:

   (a) increase respiration rates

   (b) decrease muscle tension

   (c) lower heart rate

   (d) reduce nausea

4. Acupressure as an anti-emetic:

   (a) needs trained acupuncturists to administer

   (b) must be applied to pressure points on both wrists

   (c) does not work with left-handed people

   (d) is effective even when the patient is anaesthetized

5. Guided imagery involves:
   TRUE FALSE

   (a) showing patients slides of your
       holiday

   (b) making the room smell of flowers

   (c) talking to the patient in the dark

   (d) relaxing the patient by soothing
       commentary relating to a pleasing
       image

CHAPTER 6: THE NURSING MANAGEMENT OF PATIENTS WITH NAUSEA AND VOMITING

There are a variety of situations in which the nurse will encounter a patient who is suffering from nausea and vomiting. For most situations the nausea and vomiting will be predictable – such as postoperatively or after cancer treatment. The nurse will therefore have time to plan appropriate nursing care. This chapter is a consideration of the important aspects of nursing care that deal specifically with nausea and vomiting and is aimed at defining interventions that the nurse can integrate alongside other aspects of patient care.

For patients who are in hospital with other illnesses that are accompanied by nausea and vomiting these same basic principles apply and can be adapted to the circumstances. There are fewer interventions that can be employed to alleviate the sickness associated with pregnancy or with sudden, unexpected vomiting. These situations are considered later in this chapter.

6.1 Planning nursing care

Forward planning is most easily achieved by using the nursing process. This consists of: assessing the patient's problems; defining realistic goals that will solve or alleviate the problem; planning interventions which will achieve these goals and evaluating the success of these interventions. In some units implementing this process may be a matter of being aware of this logical approach and using it as a basis for nursing care. In other units this system is used to document a formal care plan for each patient.

Two related topics that are relevant to every stage of this process and deserve further consideration are communication between the nurse and patient and patient education. A proper assessment of a patient's condition and needs is not possible if there is a lack of communication. Being able to deliver considered and accurate information is vital in helping patients understand and comply with aspects of their treatment and good communication will help a nurse provide the support that is sometimes so necessary in assisting patients though a period of serious illness.

6.2 Communication

The quality of patient-nurse communication depends on at least two things – language and willingness or ability to communicate.

There is often a problem of communication when patients use colloquial terms that the nurse might not have encountered before; or perhaps the patient does not understand the nurse's vocabulary but does not like to admit it. This seems to be particularly common when talking about nausea and vomiting. One study (from the USA) has revealed that two-thirds of hospitalized adult patients surveyed did not understand the word 'nausea' (Rhodes, *et al.*, 1984). In this case 'sick at stomach' was the more recognizable definition. The nurse and the patient therefore, must be clear that they both understand the condition that is being described; in the UK, words such as 'queasy' or 'feeling sick' are often used.

When talking to patients and their relatives it is important to distinguish between nausea, retching and vomiting in language which is mutually understood. Some of the more common colloquial terms used are summarized in Table 6.1 but there will be a number of regional variants which could be added. It may be

Table 6.1 Colloquial terms used for nausea, retching or vomiting

Nausea	Retching	Vomiting
feeling sick	heaving	throwing up
queasy	gagging	spewing
bilious	dry boak	chucking up
off colour	dry heaves	regurgitating
green at the gills		puking
under the weather		barfing
sick at stomach		chundering
		waterbrash
		being sick

useful to let patients explain their feelings in their own words and try to use the terms they find familiar.

It is particularly important to understand how a patient is using the word 'sick' and to establish that when patients say they have stopped being sick that they have also stopped feeling sick.

The broader area of ways in which nurses can facilitate patient-nurse communication is complex, and many articles and books are devoted to this topic. Only a few points can be covered here, but there are some important factors to be considered when nursing patients with nausea and vomiting.

Since nausea is a subjective sensation the nurse will often have to rely on patients to say when they are feeling unwell and need anti-emetic medication or some other intervention. Some people find it easy to ask for help and will communicate their problems to the nurse as soon as they feel discomfort. Others 'don't want to be a nuisance' and will behave stoically even though their nausea might be quite pronounced. This is obviously a reflection of the individual's personality but it is worth remembering that the patient's cultural background may influence the way they respond. Some are from cultures where public displays of distress or needing assistance are not as acceptable as in others. Some male patients may find difficulty in relating to females outside their family in anything other than a very formal way. A wider discussion of this topic is given by Sampson (1982). Acknowledgment of these differences may help the nurse adopt the most suitable approach to help the patient.

It is up to the nurse to try and facilitate communication with the patient as much as possible – given the constraints of time and the patient's own attitude. For cancer nurses, communication is particularly important. Yet, several studies have shown that cancer nurses often have a poor level of communication with their patients (see Wilkinson, 1991). Poor communication is undesirable on a number of levels, which go beyond the scope of nursing in relation to nausea and vomiting. However, a vitally important fact that emerges is that where there is a low level of communication nursing assessments of a patient's condition can be very superficial, and nursing care is subsequently based on 'little more than assumptions' (Wilkinson, 1991). This can be particularly unsatisfactory when nursing patients with nausea and vomiting. Nausea and vomiting can be exacerbated by emotional feelings – such as fear or anxiety – as well as by physical factors related to treatment and the patient's own demography. A poor assessment of the patient may not address all the causative factors that are contributing to emesis with the result that interventions are inadequate.

6.3 Patient education

Another important aspect of nursing related to communication is patient education. The majority of patients will approach their treatment with very little knowledge of what to expect. Cancer patients will often arrive with wildly exaggerated fears of how awful their treatment will be; patients about to undergo surgery will be apprehensive that they are going to feel pain or develop complications. This causes a level of fear and anxiety that can be reduced by the nurse taking time to inform the patient and his/her family what is about to happen. Reduction of stress and anxiety also reduces a patient's threshold for vomiting, making it less likely that they will be sick. Nurses are in a unique position to identify the patient's fears and worries that are often giving rise to considerable distress. Nurses spend more time than any other member of the healthcare team with patients in hospital. They often have more opportunities for communication and patients will ask questions or reveal fears to a nurse in a way that they will not to a doctor. The majority of patients who are suffering from nausea and vomiting – cancer patients and surgical patients – will be in distressing situations and nurses can fulfil an important role in patient education. Dispelling fears and misconceptions from the outset is beneficial for everybody. One author describes quite succinctly that it is the nurse's role 'to take what is foreign and fearful to the patient and make it familiar and thus less frightening' (Benner, 1984).

As relevant points of education can only be touched upon here, the reader is referred to the excellent work on this topic by Gertrud Grahn, Pat Webb and their colleagues for more information (Grahn, 1988; Grahn and Johnson, 1990; Webb, 1988), a broader discussion is given in the work edited by Webb (1994).

It is always important to establish the patient's own needs in any educative process. Patients will not assimilate complicated and detailed explanations that they do not want, and may be left with some simple questions unanswered merely because they were not given the opportunity to ask. Patients should be told what they want to know, not what the nurse thinks they ought to know.

A particularly demanding aspect of a nurse's role is to judge how much information is required by patients. This can be especially true for potential side-effects. Will describing events that may not happen produce unnecessary fears and worries in the patient? This is an important consideration in the case of nausea and vomiting – can too much concentration on side-effects precipitate vomiting, just by virtue of the anxiety created? It is tempting to think 'I shouldn't mention it in case it doesn't happen'.

In practice most nurses find that this is not the case. In fact the converse is true. It is usually found that careful explanation of side-effects leads to a better prepared patient who copes more easily with the consequences of treatment. A description of what the patient is likely to see, hear, feel, smell and taste enhance the patient's ability to cope (Strohl, 1988). In one study it was shown that the closer the description matched the actual event, the less anxiety was experienced by the patient (Johnson et al., 1978). A study which followed radiotherapy patients after treatment found that those who had received detailed descriptions of the treatment beforehand reported less disruption of their usual activities than those who were given minimal information (Johnson, et al., 1988).

Education helps to allay fears and reduce anxiety. Explanations of emesis are usually particularly welcome. When patients were asked to rate the nursing interventions which had proved most helpful in coping with emesis 'Explaining to me why I get sick' was the first or second most useful measure, surpassed only by 'Instructions what to eat and what not to eat to minimize my getting sick' (Welch, 1980). Wherever possible the patient's family or carers should be included in patient education. It is not only of practical use, but being involved can give the carers a role and help them in coming to terms with a loved one's illness.

There are likely to be constraints on how much time is available for patient education but, where possible, try to break the information down into easily assimilated units. Remember that people who are anxious and worried (this applies to carers as well as patients) can only process a small amount of information at a time. Continuing with too much explanation at one session may progressively extinguish what has gone before. A shorter explanation followed at a later opportunity by a chance to discuss what has been said previously is best. Nurses should, if possible, check that the patient has understood what has been said either at the end of a discussion or by starting the next session with a review of a previous discussion.

Oral information should be supplemented by written information whenever possible so that patients and their carers can read it at a later stage. Most cancer units provide leaflets or fact sheets. If you are nursing a patient in a non-specialist unit or such literature is scarce, there are, in most countries, support organizations that provide leaflets. The leaflets provided by Cancerlink, Bacup and the Royal Marsden Hospital are excellent (see Appendix for contact addresses).

For patients who are about to have surgery which will result in significant changes to their body – for example a colostomy, mastectomy or tracheostomy – there are often information leaflets available to help them cope with the changes.

Remember that patient education is (as is any education) an ongoing process, not a one-off event. There must be time for 'restating, clarifying and re-enforcing information as a person's capacity, desire and readiness for learning fluctuate.' (Grahn & Johnson, 1990).

6.4 Assessing the patient

The patient may already be suffering from nausea and/or vomiting before treatment starts. A distinction must be made between treatment-induced nausea and vomiting and emesis that is directly related to the patient's condition. It is important that anti-emetics are not given to any patient before the cause of the nausea and vomiting is known; symptoms could be masked before diagnosis and in some cases the vomiting is positively beneficial. For example, if vomiting is due to food poisoning it is best not to try and suppress the vomiting so that the offending material is eliminated from the body.

When nausea and vomiting are due to disease it is important that anti-emetics are not given inappropriately. Patients with gastrointestinal obstruction are not usually given anti-emetics, unless they are in palliative care. The patient should be given small, frequent drinks and observed for signs of dehydration (see section 6.8). Such patients will need urgent medical or surgical intervention.

If there are signs of nausea and vomiting due to constipation or hypercalcaemia, this should be noted.

Pain can be a contributor to nausea and vomiting and can also affect the patient's disposition. If analgesics have not been prescribed this should be discussed with the medical or surgical staff to see if better pain control can be provided at this stage.

There may be clinical reasons why analgesics cannot be given at this point.

Record the patient's weight. Make sure that the patient is not already cachexic; it may be necessary to instigate total parenteral nutrition (TPN) to bring a poorly-nourished patient into a good state for surgery.

Note any likes or dislikes for food and drinks and if a patient knows that a particular food upsets his/her digestion this should be recorded. After treatment the patient may need some encouragement to resume eating, and it is best to avoid foods that are not liked by the patient. Some patients may have special dietary requirement for medical, religious or social reasons; this should be noted.

If the patient is an out-patient or undergoing day case surgery, ask about home circumstances as the period of delayed emesis may be at its worst once they are at home. Make sure the carer is aware of the problems of nausea and vomiting or contact social services or community nurses if the patient is going to be alone at home.

People have different 'emetic thresholds' and some are far more likely to be sick than others. Establish if the patient is sick easily under other circumstances. Are they poor travellers, did they have pregnancy sickness (if appropriate), are they unable to eat spicy food?

If your unit has access to supportive techniques it might be useful to establish the patient's attitude. Some patients may benefit enormously from relaxation therapy for example, while others are sceptical and dismissive of such techniques.

If the patient has received treatment before ask how the treatment affected him/her. More obvious information will consist of what anti-emetics were given, and if they were effective. Also ask if the patients themselves have identified measures which aggravated or alleviated their condition.

Special considerations for radiotherapy and chemotherapy patients

For chemotherapy patients it is important to try and obtain the best anti-emetic control possible right from the outset. This is not only for the patient's comfort but to avoid anticipatory nausea and vomiting developing.

Controlling nausea and vomiting is usually easiest during the first session of chemotherapy, tending to become progressively harder to control as subsequent treatment courses are given. This is especially true if inadequate anti-emetic treatment was given with the first course of chemotherapy. Previous experience can provide important information for selecting future management.

The factors that predispose a patient to nausea and vomiting after radiotherapy or chemotherapy have been outlined in Chapter 3. The patient should be asked, or the relevant notes consulted, to assess the likelihood of the patient suffering from post-treatment nausea and vomiting. The chemotherapy prescribed for the patient should be checked for how emetogenic it is likely to be. Establish the patient's history of alcohol intake and factors such as susceptibility to motion sickness or pregnancy sickness should be noted.

If this is not the first course of treatment the patient should be given an opportunity to discuss if they have been experiencing delayed or anticipatory emesis. Many patients will not report anticipatory symptoms spontaneously – they think the experience means that they are behaving oddly or that the disease is affecting their mind (Morrow, 1992). Questions about anticipatory symptoms should, therefore, be included as part of routine questions and not given undue emphasis. For some patients it will be a welcome relief to learn that such symptoms are commonplace and their experience is not strange or unusual.

Some units use charts to assist in patient assessment. Such tools are useful and it may be worth producing one for your unit if there is nothing currently available. An example of an assessment tool is given in Table 6.2.

Special considerations for surgical patients

Before non-emergency surgery a patient must be prepared both emotionally and physically for an operation.

The assessment for surgical patients should include factors which predispose the patient to vomiting. These are summarized in Chapter 3 and include the site of operation, age, gender and susceptibility to other emetic stimuli. For female patients of menstrual age the date of her last menstrual period should be determined, for the phase of her cycle can influence the incidence of PONV.

If the patient has undergone surgery before, it is important to discuss past experiences. How did they react to the anaesthetic? Were there any special problems? The amount of nausea and/or vomiting they experienced as well as their attitude to the event(s) provide important information for selecting future management.

The main points to be included in the patient assessment are summarized in Table 6.3.

Table 6.2 An example of a nausea and vomiting assessment tool for chemotherapy patients. (Reprinted from the *Oncology Nursing Forum* with permission from the Oncology Nursing Press, Inc. Wickham, R. Managing Chemotherapy-related Nausea and Vomiting: the state of the art. *Oncology Nursing Forum*, **16**(14): 563–74, 1989.)

Patient . . . .
Chemotherapy regimen . . . .
Anti-emetic regimen . . . .
Have you experienced nausea/vomiting with illness, pregnancy, car sickness etc? . . . .
If so, was anything helpful to decrease this? . . . .
Have you had nausea or vomiting with past chemotherapy? . . . . .
Was this tolerable or intolerable? . . . .
What anti-nausea medicine did your doctor prescribe? . . . .
Was it helpful? . . . .
Did you take the medicine? . . . .
How often? . . . .
Did you have any side effects with the anti-nausea medicine?
. . . .
Do you think you will have vomiting from your chemotherapy?
. . . .

If the patient is receiving chemotherapy:

Are you experiencing nausea with your chemotherapy? . . . .
When does it happen (before, during, after) [onset] . . . .
How long does it last [duration] . . . .
Rate your nausea in terms of intensity . . . . and interference with your life . . . . [use a VAS scale]
Are you experiencing vomiting with your chemotherapy? . . . .
When does it happen (before, during, after) [onset] . . . .
How long does it last [duration] . . . .
Rate your vomiting in terms of intensity . . . . and interference with your life . . . . [use a VAS scale]

How satisfied are you with present control of nausea and/or vomiting? . . . .

VAS

None at all   Intolerable

0 - 10

Table 6.3   Summary of patient assessment

- Establish that there are not current problems with nausea and vomiting
- Ask about the patient's diet (likes/dislikes/food allergies)
- Establish whether the patient is prone to vomiting under other circumstances
- Make sure that the patient is not in pain
- Record the patient's weight
- Establish the patient's own expectations of treatment and perceptions of nausea and vomiting
- Discuss previous experiences
- Assess whether there are predisposing factors that will make the patient more prone to nausea and vomiting
- Contact social workers or community nurses if necessary

6.5 Nursing interventions before treatment

Having assessed the patient's risk factors and needs, check which anti-emetics have been prescribed by the physician or anaesthetists. If the anti-emetics seem inappropriate or inadequate – for example if dopamine receptor antagonists have been prescribed for children, or an overweight woman about to undergo dilatation and curettage has not been prescribed an anti-emetic, discuss this with the medical or surgical staff and note your concerns.

For day case patients, anti-emetics should be chosen with care. The patient should not be sent home feeling sedated by the medication. Oral anti-emetics should be provided for high-risk patients to take home with them.

Most anti-emetics should be given before treatment. Check the timing of administration and ensure that the dose is given appropriately. Tablets, for example, need some time to be absorbed, and while injections are usually active immediately many intravenous preparations are given by 10–15 minute infusions. Anti-emetics may be given by a variety of routes to surgical patients. For convenience tablets or intramuscular injections are given before surgery whereas infusions can be given intravenously during surgery by means of existing lines. Postoperatively the route must be appropriate. Much will depend on whether intravenous lines are present and a tablet is of little use to someone who has not resumed fluid or food intake or is actively vomiting. Remember that some anxiolytics or sedatives such as lorazepam should be prescribed and offered the night before treatment.

Special considerations for radiotherapy and chemotherapy patients

Take time to talk to the patient about their treatment. The nurse should give a brief description of the actual treatment and a rough idea of how long it will take.

Discuss how chemotherapy will be given; infusions, injections or tablets. Warn patients if any physical sensations are likely, for example if the infusion will feel cold or if they are likely to experience a warm sensation in the arm. Some patients experience a strange or metallic taste in the mouth when being given chemotherapy drugs.

Describe the time course of events. If chemotherapy is likely to produce vomiting six to eight hours later, this must be mentioned or it may come as an unwelcome shock when the patient was beginning to assume all was well.

Other side-effects, such as stomatitis, neutropenia and hair loss, should be mentioned if they are likely consequences of the patient's particular treatment regimen.

Remember that large, complicated radiotherapy apparatus can seem quite overwhelming and frightening to a patient who has not seen it before. Describe the machine or show a photograph to the patient. Radiotherapy patients have been shown to be concerned about being left alone in the treatment room and have fears that the machine may crush them. Because radiation cannot be seen, patients fear that they will receive too much or be burned by the rays (Bricourt & McKenzie, 1984). All these fears will be reduced if the nurse has explained the process of radiotherapy treatment in detail.

Radiotherapy-induced vomiting may not occur until a week or two into the treatment schedule. Radiotherapy also can produce fatigue which tends to appear, or become worse, around the third or fourth week of treatment. Patients who are unprepared for this often perceive the fatigue as a sign that treatment is ineffective and worry that the cancer is progressing (Strohl, 1988).

Chemotherapy should be given in a relaxed unhurried atmosphere and this is often a good time to discuss any problems the patient may be having.

There is not always room for flexibility in scheduling treatment sessions. However, when it is possible avoid obviously unsuitable times such as mealtimes. Try to arrange that patients who are going home will not be travelling during the period when they are at most risk of vomiting, or are sedated.

Radiotherapy patients may have less vomiting when treated at midday or in the afternoon than when treated in the morning (Welch, 1980). Whether the time of day that chemotherapy is given has any effect on the amount of vomiting has been studied (Headley, 1987) but no significant differences occurred when the patients received chemotherapy in the morning (06.00 to 12.00 noon) or the evening (18.00–24.00). Patients treated in the evening tended to experience fewer emetic episodes and 'less distress'. However, as the authors themselves concede, this may be due to the fact that the night-time environment is less stimulating. Influential factors may be the absence of food odours and stressful situations and sleep may overcome mild nausea. (Remember some anti-emetics act by virtue of sedating the patient).

If the anti-emetics are likely to cause sedation it may cause less inconvenience if they are given later in the day.

Special considerations for surgical patients

For elective surgery food and drink should be withheld from the patient for at least six hours before surgery (see Pritchard & Mallett, 1992). Research has shown that patients often did not understand why they were deprived of food or drink (Thomas, 1987) so it is worthwhile taking a few moments to explain this.

The surgeon will probably have already explained the operation to the patient and this may not be the time for lengthy discussions of the patient's condition. But it is helpful to tell the patient what to expect in the next few hours.

An unsuspecting patient who recovers from the anaesthetic to find an intravenous infusion, cannula, drain or urinary catheter in place may be very frightened. Telling the patient beforehand to expect the presence of these items will do much to relieve anxiety.

The majority of patients will have little idea of how they will feel as the anaesthetic wears off and a few minutes spent describing the sensations can do much to alleviate unwarranted fears.

It is not uncommon to taste or smell the anaesthetic, especially as one exhales. This may precipitate feelings of nausea. Most patients have a dry mouth – due to the use of anti-sialagogues – and, especially if an airway has been inserted, the throat will be uncomfortable or sore. Some patients feel 'bloated'. Those who have undergone abdominal surgery may

Table 6.4 Nursing interventions before treatment

- Make sure the patient understands what treatment they are about to receive
- Explain the nature and likely time course of treatment sessions
- Explain the nature and timing of side-effects
- Be realistic, but not alarmist, about the possibility of nausea and vomiting occurring
- Explain the measures that will alleviate nausea and vomiting – identify the patient's own preferences
- Inform the patient that anti-emetics are available
- Check that suitable anti-emetics have been prescribed

have had the abdomen distended by carbon dioxide, which produces feelings of abdominal 'fullness' and the surprising sensation of aches and/or pains around the shoulders. There will be special considerations for certain types of surgery – for example the presence of traction, colostomy bags etc. – and these should be discussed.

The fact that patients may feel very cold or awake feeling nauseous should be discussed. Patients should be told to inform the nursing staff if they feel nauseous.

These factors are summarized in table 6.4.

6.6 Nursing interventions after treatment

Remember that emetic stimuli are cumulative or additive. Different factors can build up feelings of nausea or stimulate different emetic pathways until some threshold is reached and the patient starts to vomit. So keeping precipitating factors to a minimum helps patient comfort.

After treatment – radiotherapy, chemotherapy or the surgical procedure – make the patient as comfortable as possible in a bed or chair. The surgical patient will be lying down, most patients are more comfortable lying on their side. Move patients slowly and as they recover avoid sitting them 'bolt upright' too soon as this can cause a drop in blood pressure that may induce feelings of nausea. For patients who have undergone surgery of the throat, make sure there is no blood in the throat as this can irritate the oesophagus. Children who have had adeno-tonsillectomy should be placed lying on one side with the head lowered (lateral decubitus position) (Lerman, 1992). Be aware that sometimes after surgery a recumbent patient may be feeling well enough to attempt getting out of bed but the postural hypotension caused by this manoeuvre may bring on feelings of nausea quite suddenly – especially if the movement is accompanied by pain.

Position vulnerable patients away from strong odours or very public places. Consider who will be in the neighbouring bed; the sight and sounds of fellow patients who are coughing up sputum, who have fungating wounds, diarrhoea or who are vomiting themselves can be very distressing. These sights and sounds may be enough of an emetic stimulus to precipitate vomiting in your patient. Patients with advanced cancer are particularly sensitive to smells.

Most important, and often forgotten, is to have a receiver and tissues to hand but preferably out of sight as they can act as a stimulus and precipitate vomiting.

Avoid leaning over the patient and exhaling bad breath – last night's garlic or the odour of cigarettes are often unpleasant and can precipitate nausea. Even perfume or aftershave that may appeal to the wearer can be overpowering especially in the recovery room.

Visitors should be encouraged not to introduce strong odours such as those mentioned above. Similarly highly perfumed gifts, such as soaps and perfumed cards, may upset some patients.

Most patients find being sick in public quite embarrassing. Be sensitive to their feelings; reassure them that it is quite acceptable to be sick; provide screens or privacy if possible.

While appreciating privacy from the general public many patients will want to have a nurse at hand when they are vomiting. Ask if there are any interventions that help them feel better – for example a damp flannel for the patient's forehead. The amount of contact and assistance the nurse can provide will depend very much on individual circumstances.

Following a period of vomiting most patients will want to wash their hands and face. If the patient is unable to do so, or is not fully recovered from the anaesthetic, some assistance may be appreciated. If appropriate a mouthwash should be provided. Some mouthwashes, especially those containing chlorhexidine, have strong tastes or smells that might best be avoided in this situation. Alcohol-containing preparations are not recommended as they can increase the dryness of the mouth, which is unpleasant and damaging to the mucosa. In these circumstances water may be sufficient to rinse the mouth.

After surgery vomiting may be unproductive but patients will still appreciate moistening their mouth. Mouthwashes should not be used after oral surgery or adenotonsillectomy unless they have been indicted by the surgeon.

Oral hygiene is important not only for patient comfort but also to prevent medical complications. Many cytotoxic drugs cause stomatitis; affected areas will not only be painful but can become infected, especially by species of Candida. This is not only unpleasant but, in the immunocompromised or severely debilitated patient, such infections become established quite rapidly and can enter the systemic circulation.

After vomiting has occurred any soiled bed linen should be removed as quickly as possible not only for the comfort of the patient but the odour may permeate the rest of the ward or room, causing other patients to feel nauseous. The usual precautions for handling body fluids should be employed, bearing in mind that if a patient vomits soon after receiving oral chemotherapy then cytotoxic agents may be present in the vomitus.

After surgery it will take time for fluid and food intake to be resumed. When sips of water are allowed these must be restricted to small sips; gulping water may precipitate vomiting.

A patient feeling nauseous may benefit from sipping iced water or a fizzy drink through a straw. Ginger is a long-standing remedy for all sorts of gastric disturbances and ginger ale is often recommended for helping to relieve feelings of nausea. Dry crackers or toast can help.

Most patients will not want to eat if they are feeling at all sick and it is best to avoid strong food aromas by discrete positioning of food trolleys. There is little information published on how dietary adjustments help to control nausea and vomiting. Scogna and Smalley (1979) suggest that for chemotherapy patients it makes little difference, although those receiving radiotherapy had less problems when they ate a large meal before treatment and had only light meals throughout the rest of the day.

Those patients who can face food are still vulnerable to emetogenic stimuli and some thought should be given to the meal they are offered. Presentation is important, however, and removing the plate cover and allowing the more pungent odours to dissipate before giving the meal to the patient helps. Small, frequent snacks are usually better received than large meals. Carbohydrate is usually more acceptable and spicy or fatty foods should be avoided. Fats slow gastric emptying and will add to any feelings of nausea.

There is some evidence that fluid intake can affect the amount of vomiting (Jordan, 1989); patients who are dehydrated or who drank more than 1000 ml of water during treatment suffered more emesis than those who were in normal fluid balance and maintained a moderate intake (400–1000 ml).

Pain is an emetic stimulus and it seems a particular injustice for some patients that the analgesic given (opioids for example) may control the pain but produces nausea and vomiting! If this is the case then anti-emetics must be given with or, preferably, before the analgesic. Talk to the patient and try to ensure that they are not failing to ask for pain relief for fear of feeling nauseated when it is administered. A summary of post-treatment interventions is given in Table 6.5.

Special considerations for surgical patients

The nursing care required in the recovery room after a surgical procedure is highly specialized. The patient will be under close observation at all times and looking for signs of nausea and or vomiting will be part of these observations. Any patient who is vomiting before regaining consciousness must be turned on one side with the head down and the mouth evacuated. If necessary suction should be used and the patient may require oxygen (see Pritchard & Mallett, 1992). If the patient's jaws have been wired then the location of wire cutters should be known in case of an emergency.

When the patient is moved from the recovery room to the

Table 6.5   Summary of nursing interventions after treatment

- Make the patient comfortable in bed or a chair
- Move patients slowly; motion, postural hypotension and pain all contribute to feelings of nausea and vomiting
- Consider where the patient is to be located on the ward
- Avoid strong odours; food, perfume etc.
- Provide privacy
- Have receivers and tissues discretely located
- Provide washing facilities
- Pay attention to oral hygiene
- Change bed linen promptly
- Offer cold water or fizzy drinks
- Check anti-emetics and ensure that they are being given appropriately

ward the general considerations discussed above are applicable there are also some other factors which are especially pertinent to the surgical patient.

If appropriate, pressure should be applied to the wound during retching and vomiting to reduce strain and discomfort. This is especially true for abdominal wounds. Help the patient to do this or tell them that pressure is useful.

Patients undergoing elective surgery will have been fasted for six hours and should have an empty stomach. For surgical emergencies it is necessary to aspirate the stomach contents. This may not be totally effective and such patients should be closely observed for signs of vomiting as vomitus can block airways or cause aspiration pneumonia. When the patient has resumed spontaneous breathing the airway should be removed to avoid stimulating the pharyngeal pathways and the 'gag' response.

If any anti-emetics were given pre-operatively or during the operation the dose and timing should be noted, and if a subsequent dose has been prescribed it should be ready and given at the correct time. Adhering to the schedule is particularly important for patients in whom it is imperative to avoid vomiting.

If anti-emetics are to be given as required then the patient should be observed for the first signs of nausea (pallor, sweating) or retching. If conscious the patient should be asked if he or she feels nauseous.

6.7 Monitoring the patient

Make sure that appropriate anti-emetics have been prescribed for the days following treatment. Some anti-emetics are given prophylactically to prevent nausea and vomiting, others are prescribed to treat the problem when it occurs. The nurse should be aware of which strategy has been employed for the particular patient being nursed. Repeat doses of anti-emetics should be ready and given at the correct time. If anti-emetics are to be given on a PRN basis then the patient should be informed that anti-emetics are available.

If the prescribed anti-emetic is clearly ineffective then this should be discussed with the medical or surgical staff as soon as possible. The anti-emetic regimen can usually be changed or extra drugs given.

If vomiting is a continual problem for a chemotherapy patient it may be possible to change the chemotherapy regimen. This may mean changing the drugs or may be achieved by altering doses or routes of administration. With experience the nurse may be able to identify the offending cytotoxic drug and discuss this with the medical staff. The nurse should explain to the patient that, if one course of therapy is particularly unpleasant, there are changes that can be made to make the next course more tolerable.

It is interesting to note that several years ago (1986) a survey of cancer nurses' attitudes revealed that nurses found it very stressful to care for cancer patients as they thought the patients were being over-treated – a conclusion based on the incidence and severity of side-effects, notably nausea and vomiting, that they witnessed. As anti-emetic control has improved, the introduction of 5-HT$_3$ receptor antagonists being a major innovation, a follow-up study, in 1993, has shown that nurses no longer find nursing chemotherapy patients so stressful. Sixty six (88%) of the nurses mentioned that this was due to improved anti-emetic regimens which had contributed to patient care. Perhaps not surprisingly in the current climate the source of stress had shifted to hospital under-resourcing and inadequate levels of staffing (Wilkinson, 1994).

When nausea and vomiting are persistent the patient must be closely observed for signs of dehydration. The patient's fluid balance should be monitored. Accurate records of intravenous infusions and oral fluids should be made and all fluid loss recorded. For surgical patients this includes loss by wound or stoma drainage, nasogastric drainage, vomitus and urine. Signs of dehydration are covered in section 6.8.

6.8 Dehydration

Patients who are vomiting for prolonged periods (especially cancer patients) are in danger of becoming dehydrated.

Dehydration can range from a very mild condition, which can be averted by early intervention, to more severe situations when intravenous fluids are required. It is difficult to make generalizations but the majority of cancer and postoperative patients will probably need some intravenous fluids. Fluid intake must be monitored and if possible the volume of liquid produced on vomiting should be recorded. A good fluid balance is also necessary to avoid the nephrotoxic effects of some cytotoxic drugs, especially cisplatinum. It is important, therefore, to see that patients are offered frequent drinks.

Postoperative patients are in a catabolic state and the daily fluid requirement is about 30 ml/kg/day (Shearer & Hunter, 1992). Intravenous fluid will need to be maintained until the patient can tolerate this volume of fluid by mouth.

Mild dehydration is not easily recognized; there are few outward signs and blood pressure remains normal until an advanced stage. The initial signs of dehydration are thirst and a dry tongue, but a patient who is feeling nauseated may be unable to face a drink in spite of suffering these effects.

As dehydration progresses urine output decreases with a resultant rise in its specific gravity. Continued dehydration will cause a furrowed tongue, decreased turgidity of the skin, difficulty in swallowing, mental confusion, elevated blood urea and electrolytes. Table 6.6 provides a summary of the signs of dehydration.

The most convenient parameter that can be measured is the specific gravity of urine – this can often be done on the ward. If dehydration is suspected the medical staff should be informed so that blood samples can be taken for urea and electrolyte measurements.

Electrolytes are also lost along with fluid when vomiting occurs. The most common electrolyte imbalance seen in patients with severe vomiting is loss of hydrogen and chloride ions, giving rise to metabolic alkalosis. The signs of alkalosis are shallow, slow respiration, irregular pulse and muscle cramps. Metabolic alkalosis can cause a patient to appear irritable and unco-operative.

Persistent nausea can also impinge on a patient's progress by causing depression and loss of morale. Nurses will then need to provide some level of emotional or psychological support to their patients.

6.9 Psychological support

Although situations will differ the nurse, in conjunction with the patient's family and friends, will probably be the mainstay of the support provided to the patient. The balance will shift depending on whether the patient is in or out of hospital or is receiving care in other environments, such as a hospice. The patient's family may also look to the nurse for information and support.

When people are ill, particularly if they are receiving hospital treatment, they often experience feelings of helplessness and being overwhelmed by their disease, or the environment their

Table 6.6 Symptoms relating to the loss of body fluid

Loss of total body fluid	Symptom or clinical manifestation
1%–2%	Thirst
Mild-moderate dehydration	
2%–5%	Dryness of tongue
	Scanty or decreased urine output
	High urine specific gravity
	Furrowed tongue
	Decreased turgidity of skin
5%–8%	Elevated BUN
	Fatigue
	Increased pulse
	Elevated temperature
	Deterioration of mental processes
Serious dehydration	
6%–8%	Protein, casts and erythrocytes excreted in urine
	Loss of skin turgor
Severe dehydration	
8%–10%	Sunken eyeballs
	Profound depression
	Anuria
	10% increase in haematocrit
11%–15%	Delirium
	Deafness
	Kidney failure
10%–20%	Death

(Table modified from: Carpenter, L. (1987) *Dehydration and Symptom Distress During Cancer Chemotherapy*, unpublished master's thesis. Given in Nolan, 1985.)

disease places them in. This can be relieved, in part, by involving patients in their own treatment. Part of the success of some supportive techniques is because patients feel that they are gaining some control over their situation. Such feelings can be encouraged by nurses establishing a partnership situation where the patient and nurse together define strategies for coping with the illness or the side-effects. Treating emesis lends itself particularly well to this approach as there can be a high degree of flexibility in anti-emetic therapy. Different types of anti-emetic drugs are available and supportive therapies can be used alongside more conventional regimens.

Support for cancer patients

Continuity of care in cancer nursing is vital as patients build up a dependence and trust in the nurses caring for them. It is possible that, in some situations the nurse can be a 'cue' to anticipatory nausea and vomiting. The nurse and patient together must then establish whether the anticipatory symptoms outweigh the benefits of knowing the nurse who will be providing care.

For patients being treated in an out-patient setting, seeing the same nurse for every cycle of therapy not only has psychological benefits but allows a better assessment of their physical condition and morale and thus a more thorough documentation of toxicities. The nurse is also more likely to notice if a patient is postponing appointments. A reluctance to comply with treatment schedules may be a sign that the patient is experiencing severe nausea and vomiting and/or is developing anticipatory symptoms.

Some patients however may not want to talk about their problems. In a study where 79% of the patients were experiencing nausea and vomiting, only 33% said they would mention this to the doctor (Welch, 1980) – how many would mention it to a nurse was not specified, but it does show a reluctance to communicate problems. Nurses cannot force communication and must respect the patient's own opinion.

There will be situations where the nurse alone cannot cope with a patient's particular problem, and with the patient's consent, may have to call on extra support to assist the patient through a course of treatment. A therapist specialized in supportive techniques may help or the assistance of a clinical psychologist or psychiatrist may be necessary. In such cases the introduction of other professionals must not be regarded as disturbing the nurse/patient relationship. The entire healthcare team can act in a co-ordinated manner to achieve the best possible care and support for the patient and under such circumstances the nurse may play a crucial role in co-ordinating team efforts.

A multi-disciplinary approach may be especially useful when a patient refuses further treatment. This is not a common occurrence but can happen, even when the patient appears to be coping well. This is distressing, but it is important for the nurse not to feel personally slighted by the patient's attitude or take it as a reflection of the quality of care delivered. The nurse must remain calm and keep a sense of perspective; help from colleagues must be sought.

6.10 Instructing out-patients or patients being discharged

Patients must be aware that nausea and vomiting can occur for days or even weeks after some radio- or chemotherapy. Good anti-emetic control on the day of treatment does not necessarily mean continuing freedom from emesis, so patients should be warned of potential problems.

Delayed emesis is not so problematic after surgery but some patients will experience nausea for several days and where there has been gastrointestinal involvement feelings of nausea, dyspepsia or indigestion may persist.

Most patients will have been told about measures to alleviate nausea during their treatment. This information should be reiterated. If anti-emetics are being supplied it is important the patient understands how and when they should be taken. Continuing contact with the patient will vary depending on your unit or your country. Any continuing care should be organized before the patient is discharged and arrangements made for the effectiveness of anti-emetics to be included in the review of the patient's progress. Written information is essential for the patient to take home (see Table 6.7).

In many countries there are support organizations for patients who have undergone certain types of surgery. Such organizations are usually for patients whose operation has made a major change in their lifestyle; for example tracheostomy or colostomy. These groups generally provide practical help as well as emotional support and the patient should be introduced to useful organizations (see Appendix for further information).

The information given in these preceding sections has been summarized in Table 6.8.

6.11 Women with pregnancy sickness

Following the sad experiences of fetal malformations due to drugs taken in pregnancy, the administration of any medication to a pregnant woman – especially in the first trimester – is avoided. Many pregnant women, but by no means all, feel sick

Table 6.7 Information for patients being discharged or receiving out-patient treatment

- Make sure the patient is informed about the likely pattern of nausea and vomiting
- Explain how and when anti-emetic medication should be taken
- Warn the patient if anti-emetics are likely to cause sedation
- Ensure that carer understands this information
- Outline the methods used to relieve nausea – even if this has been done before
- Help the patient to identify precipitating factors and ways of avoiding these
- Emphasize the need to maintain adequate food and fluid intake
- Provide dietary suggestion leaflets/recipe sheets for light meals
- During subsequent hospital visits look for signs of dehydration or poor nutrition
- Discuss anticipatory symptoms
- Provide written information if possible and ensure that the patient's family or friends have access to useful leaflets and information
- Make sure the patient is aware of appropriate support groups

first thing in the morning. Simple dietary measures often help. Many women find that avoiding coffee, drinking weak tea or water and eating crackers, dry biscuits or dry toast relieves the nausea. The metabolic demands of being pregnant are considerable and pregnant women should not go for long periods without food as hypoglycaemia can cause nausea.

Pregnant women are best advised to try non-pharmacological therapy for nausea and vomiting and acupressure (Dundee, 1988) and aromatherapy have proved useful. They should be reassured that vomiting is not harmful and does not adversely affect the outcome of the pregnancy.

If nausea and vomiting are severe and seriously compromising nutritional intake, more drastic measures are needed. High calorie food supplements may be necessary and frequent small meals may be more acceptable.

Persistent and frequent vomiting – *hyperemesis gravidarum* – requires medical attention. In such cases the severity and consequences of the vomiting may outweigh the reluctance to prescribe medication and anti-emetics may have to be given under medical supervision.

Table 6.8 Summary of strategies for nursing patients with treatment-induced nausea and vomiting

Patient problem	Nursing aim	Nursing intervention	Rationale
Patient anxious about nausea and vomiting before treatment has started	• To alleviate anxiety • To reduce the probability of vomiting occurring	• Take time to explain treatment. Explain about nausea and vomiting • Reassure that vomiting is not inevitable but be realistic about the likelihood of it occurring • Inform the patient that anti-emetics will be available	• Anxiety can precipitate vomiting, reducing anxiety through education and reassurance will help the patient to be prepared and thus cope better
Patient feels nauseous but is acting stoically	• To identify nausea in a patient even when there is no verbal communication. • To alleviate the nausea	• Ask how the patient is feeling. Use vocabulary familiar to the patient • Give sips of fizzy drinks/dry crackers • Remove any exacerbating factors • Review the patient's anti-emetic status	• Patients are usually only stoical about mild nausea. Severe nausea is less easily tolerated and more apparent to an observer. Intervention at this stage can circumvent more serious problems
Patient feels very nauseous	• To relieve nausea • To prepare (discreetly) for the patient to vomit	• Make the patient's bed or chair comfortable or move patient if necessary • Try to increase privacy – for example screens • Try to soothe/relax the patient by contact, verbal comments, music or other techniques as appropriate to your unit • Give fizzy drink/dry crackers • Remove exacerbating factors • Reassure patient that vomiting is acceptable • Locate receiver/tissues discreetly. Place these within reach of the patient if necessary • Review the patient's anti-emetic status	• Anxiety is a contributory factor to nausea.Lowering patient's stress will help relieve the nausea • Sometimes vomiting is inevitable so making the patient feel prepared may be the only really helpful intervention • Anti-emetics may relieve the situation
• Patient is vomiting	• To assist patient through the event with the minimum of disruption, distress or embarrassment	• Provide screens if appropriate • Provide receiver or suitable receptacle • Assure patient that it is not an unusual or unacceptable occurrence • Use physical contact if appropriate, hold the patient's hand or shoulders or wipe the brow • Review anti-emetic prescription	• Practical care and emotional support must be the first priority. Anti-emetics should be reviewed as soon as possible after vomiting has stopped

Table 6.8 *Continued*

Patient problem	Nursing aim	Nursing intervention	Rationale
Patient has just stopped vomiting	• To make patient as comfortable as possible	• Place patient in most comfortable position • Remove receivers and soiled tissues • Change any soiled linen • Provide facilities for washing, at least face and hands • Give mouthwash if appropriate • Review anti-emetic prescription. If vomiting has occurred despite recent medication consider increasing dose or frequency, addition of further agents to initial anti-emetic or changing medication • Report problem to medical staff • Consider complementary techniques • Review fluid/food intake of patient	• Possible that anti-emetics are not being administered correctly • Anti-emetics currently prescribed may not be suitable for this patient/treatment
Patient vomiting frequently	• To control vomiting	• Review anti-emetic prescription • Discuss with medical staff • Try to identify any exacerbating factors and remove them • Consider complementary techniques • Review fluid balance and nutritional status of patient • Set up fluid balance chart if one is not in operation • Contact dietician, if appropriate	• Possible that anti-emetics are not being administered correctly • Anti-emetic currently prescribed may not be suitable for this patient/treatment
Patient showing signs of dehydration	• To maintain patient in normal fluid balance	• Check specific gravity of urine • Review fluid balance chart • Offer drinks frequently • Report any signs or symptoms to medical staff • Discuss requirements for iv fluids with medical staff • Contact dietician, if necessary	• Dehydration can cause medical complications and early intervention is vital • Frequent drinks may circumvent the problem. iv fluids are given routinely with (or before) several cytotoxic drugs

Table 6.8 *Continued*

Patient problem	Nursing aim	Nursing intervention	Rationale
Patient shows signs of electrolyte imbalance	• To maintain patient in normal electrolyte balance	• Report any signs or symptoms to medical staff • Check plasma electrolytes or ensure medical staff have done so • Ensure adequate diet/dietary supplements are given	• Electrolyte imbalance can cause medical complications. Early intervention is necessary

(For radiotherapy and chemotherapy patients)

Patient problem	Nursing aim	Nursing intervention	Rationale
Patient is developing anticipatory symptoms	• To prevent or reduce anticipatory symptoms	• Establish that anticipatory symptoms are occurring • Consult patient and family/friends to minimize contact with 'cues' that exacerbate the condition. (Remember some patients prefer to see the same nurse for treatment, even when the nurse is the cue) • Consider supportive techniques • Discuss the problem with other members of the oncology team	• Anticipatory symptoms respond poorly to anti-emetic drugs. Psychological support and complementary techniques may be more helpful
Patient is cancelling appointments and delaying treatment	• To assist patient to adhere to the optimum schedule of treatment	• Discuss problem with patient and/or family and friends • Establish that the patient understands the importance of the treatment schedule • Try to ascertain if anticipatory symptoms of fear of nausea and vomiting are responsible. Discuss changes to schedule that may help	• Patient may not realize the importance of the timing of treatment or not be aware that treatment is being delayed • Anticipatory symptoms may be the problem but the patient is reluctant to volunteer such information, regarding this as a 'strange' response to treatment
Patient is refusing further treatment	• To establish that this is a considered decision on the part of the patient • To assist the patient in continuing therapy, if this is appropriate	• Discuss reasons for non-compliance with patient • Enlist support from family, friends, medical staff and psychologists or psychiatrists	• Non-compliance may be a short-lived reaction to a particularly unpleasant episode or may be a considered decision on the part of the patient. It is essential to distinguish between the two. Depending on prognosis and patient's reaction the nurse must assist the patient to continue treatment or not. Ultimately it is the patient's decision

Table 6.8 *Continued*

Patient problem	Nursing aim	Nursing intervention	Rationale
(For surgical patients)			
Patient has just been moved from theatre to recovery room	• To assess risk of vomiting for this patient • To ensure that vomiting does not present a hazard while the patient is very drowsy	• Check patient's notes to assess the risk • Observe the patient closely during the risk period • Check if anti-emetics have been given and ensure that suitable anti-emetics are available	• By being aware of risk factors particularly vulnerable patients may be identified • Aspiration of voitus or gastric acid is a hazard

6.12 Patients presenting with unexpected and/or violent vomiting

Violent episodes of vomiting that start unexpectedly and have no immediately obvious cause in the patient's eyes, may be very frightening for a patient, especially if there is blood in the vomitus (haematemesis).

Such vomiting can be a symptom of a serious underlying condition and, although these situations are rare, it is of paramount importance to establish the cause of the vomiting and whether it is serious and requires urgent medical intervention.

Anti-emetics should never be given to patients if the cause of the nausea and vomiting is not known.

Nausea and vomiting that is due to a serious underlying pathology will usually be accompanied by other symptoms. Table 6.9 is a guide to attendant symptoms and possible causes. In all cases medical attention should be sought urgently.

There are conditions which are not so urgent and may not need immediate emergency treatment but nevertheless require prompt medical intervention.

If common causes such as food poisoning or infection are not suspected, the patient is not reacting to medication and has no obvious gastrointestinal problem then the nausea and vomiting could be due to migraine or ear disorders, vertigo or Ménière's disease.

Continued and persistent vomiting that is not violent can also be indicative of a serious disease condition, for example cancer of the pancreas. Patients with prolonged vomiting must always be seen by a doctor.

Table 6.9 Vomiting suggestive of serious conditions

Attendant symptoms	Possible cause
Abdominal pain not relieved by vomiting	Serious abdominal condition: perforated ulcer appendicitis
Haematemesis (red blood may be present or the vomitus will have a 'coffee grounds' appearance)	Mallory-Weiss tear of the oesophagus/gastric cardia. Bleeding elsewhere in the upper gastrointestinal tract
Headache After trauma	If a head injury has occurred within the last 24 hours this could be a sign of brain damage
Without trauma associated with sensitivity to light drowsiness confusion	Meningitis Sub-arachnoid haemorrhage
Stiff neck Sensitivity to light	Meningitis
Pain in or around one eye and blurred vision	Acute glaucoma – more likely in patients over 40 years old
Sudden forceful vomiting without nausea Headache which is worse on lying down	Raised intracranial pressure – encephalitis

6.13 Concluding remarks

The nursing needs of a patient experiencing nausea and vomiting will depend very much on the underlying physical and physiological conditions giving rise to the problem. Probably the majority of situations in which patients are suffering from nausea and vomiting are following surgery and when undergoing cancer treatment. Close attention to the patient's condition, anti-emetic drugs and well considered nursing intervention can do much to resolve the problem and bring relief.

Symptom control is an aspect of healthcare that is falling increasingly into the domain of the nurse. It is vital, therefore, that the nurse has the knowledge and skills to respond to the patient experiencing nausea and vomiting with confidence.

Summary of Chapter 6

- Nursing a patient who is suffering nausea and vomiting presents a variety of challenges. Providing effective anti-emetic control adds to the patient's quality of life.
- In some circumstances vomiting may be indicative of a serious pathological condition and nurses should be aware of this.
- Where nausea and vomiting are predictable nursing strategies must be planned in advance. It is often helpful to involve the patient in such planning.
- The nurse must assess the patient and take time to educate the patient and other relevant carers.
- Nursing strategies should consist of: assessment; planning interventions; implementing intervention and evaluating how well they are working.
- The nurse must monitor how nausea and vomiting are impinging on her/his patient's progress and evaluate whether emetic control is successful.
- Psychological support is essential.
- Other healthcare professionals may be needed and the nurse should play a central role in enlisting their support and co-ordinating their efforts.
- Pharmacologically active substances should be avioded during the first trimester of pregnancy.
- Patients with sudden unexpected and/or forceful nausea and vomiting are rare, but usually require urgent treatment.

1. Rate the following statements as true or false:

	TRUE	FALSE
(a) patients should not be told about treatment-related symptoms as this can produce nausea and vomiting		
(b) descriptions of what is about to happen during treatment will frighten most patients and should be avoided		
(c) anti-emetics should not be given before surgery because their effect will wear off too soon		

2. The following may be a stimulus for a patient to begin vomiting:

(a) smell of food		
(b) sound of another patient vomiting		
(c) sight of the chemotherapy drugs		
(d) entering the hospital		

3. Chemotherapy should be administered:

(a) in a quiet, relaxed atmosphere		
(b) as quickly as possible		
(c) somewhere busy to provide distraction		

4. Are the following true or false?

	TRUE	FALSE

(a) vomit receivers should be prominently placed on any ward where patients are likely to suffer from nausea and vomiting

(b) a nurse must be in attendance when a patient is vomiting

(c) all chemotherapy drugs cause vomiting two hours after administration

(d) chemotherapy must be administered by different members of staff each time to prevent anticipatory nausea and vomiting

(e) after surgery patients should not be sat bolt upright

5. Dehydration:

(a) can be assessed by measuring specific gravity of urine

(b) is not serious when at the 6–10% level

(c) does not cause changes in electrolytes

(d) is not a problem after surgery if the patient is able to drink

QUESTIONS FOR DISCUSSION

1. Adequate control of nausea and vomiting relies on efficient assessment of the patient and a thorough understanding of the causative factors. What as a nurse can you do to facilitate communication and assessment of the patient?

2. List the points you would consider important to assess before a patient undergoes treatment that is likely to produce nausea and vomiting.

3. 'A little knowledge is a dangerous thing'. Discuss this idea in relation to educating patients about nausea and vomiting.

4. A patient with testicular teratoma, whom you know well, arrives in the ward for his third course of chemotherapy. He is obviously distressed and states, quite adamantly, that he is not going to have any further treatment. How would you deal with this?

5. You have a patient in your ward who has received 12 of a course of 20 fractions of radiotherapy to her upper abdomen. She is persistently nauseated and has poor dietary intake. What problems is this patient likely to develop? What measures can you take to minimize them?

6. A patient is receiving chemotherapy on five consecutive days. On day 3 this patient starts to vomit. Can you establish whether this is acute vomiting due to treatment on day 3, delayed vomiting from day 2 or vomiting in anticipation of the treatment to come on day 4? Does it actually matter? Would your responses and nursing strategies change if you could identify the type of vomiting?

7. Mrs S., a 32 year old woman is married with two children aged four and six. Her husband travels regularly on business and is often away during the week. Mrs S. has breast cancer and is to receive three weekly chemotherapy courses with cyclophosphamide, adriamycin and 5-fluorouracil. Discuss the emetogenicity of this chemotherapy regimen and the implications for Mrs S. when at home.

8. Mrs D., a 46 year old woman, divorced with three children aged 22, 20 and 16 has breast cancer. She is receiving chemotherapy on an out-patient basis (cyclophosphamide, methotrexate and 5-fluorouracil). She has developed

anticipatory nausea and vomiting after one course of chemotherapy. Discuss ways of helping this patient to cope with her problem.

9. A 69 year old widower living alone has been diagnosed as having lung cancer. He is to receive chemotherapy as an in-patient in the hospital – a five day course every four weeks – that will include carboplatin, ifosfamide, mesna and eto-poside. Discuss the potential problems that may be encountered in caring for this patient with reference to chemotherapy-induced nausea and vomiting.

10. Mrs C. is a 45 year old woman with three children who is being prepared for a hysterectomy. What information about emesis would you impart to your patient?

11. A young boy arrives on the ward for strabismus repair sur-gery. What would you tell him and what would you tell his parents about the operation?

12. An elderly gentleman is to undergo a colostomy. He lives alone. What would you do to assist his recovery?

13. A woman is ten weeks pregnant and vomiting daily. She is concerned that the physical exertion of vomiting will harm her baby and so tries to avoid eating. What would you do to help this lady?

14. A young mother contacts you because her baby vomits after every feed. What further information would you like before you suggest the next course of action?

15. A terminally ill patient with gastrointestinal obstruction has been prescribed metoclopramide, which is not helping. Are you surprised? What alternative drugs would you suggest?

GLOSSARY

ACCS   Analogue continuous chromatic scale.

afferent   An afferent nerve conducts impulses from the periphery to the central nervous system.

agonist   An agent which acts on a receptor to produce a response, which is similar to the normal action of that receptor.

alkalosis   Disturbance of homeostatic mechanisms such that the plasma has an alkaline pH (around 7.5).

amine   A molecule containing a NH_2 group (ammonia is NH_3).

amino acid   A molecule that contains an amino and a COOH (carboxyl) group. Amino acids are the building blocks of protein molecules.

antagonist   An agent which acts on a receptor to block the normal response caused by stimulating that receptor.

antisialogogue   Drug which inhibits saliva secretion.

anxiolytic   A drug which reduces anxiety.

AP   The area postrema, a bilateral structure on the floor of the IV ventricle containing the CTZ.

autonomic   The autonomic nervous system controls body functions which are carried out unconsciously – for example breathing, digestion.

BBB   Blood-brain barrier.

bio-availability The percentage of a drug that is biologically available – that is the amount that is absorbed and passes into the bloodstream. When a drug is administered i.v. it is 100% bio-available.

blood-brain barrier	A functional barrier between blood and brain achieved by relatively impermeable capillaries.
bradycardia	Slow heart rate.
cerebral cortex	The outermost, largest and most highly evolved part of the brain.
CNS	Central nervous system.
cortex	Outermost layer.
CSF	Cerebro-spinal fluid.
CTZ	Chemoreceptor trigger zone.
cytotoxic	Poisonous to living cells.
dopamine	A neurotransmitter; chemically it is an amine: 3-hydroxytyramine.
dysphoria	Disturbed mood.
dystonia	Unco-ordinated movement.
enterochromaffin cell	Cells of the gastric mucosa which contain large amounts of 5-HT (*Gk entero* = gut; *chromaffin* = colour loving i.e. easily stained in histological preparations).
EPR	Extrapyramidal reaction.
extrapyramidal reaction	Lack of control of certain muscular movements.
extrapyramidal system	Complex nervous pathways involved in regulation of muscle tone, posture and stereotyped movement.
Gray	The unit used to measure radiation. This is the delivered dose.
5-HIAA	5-hydroxyindole acetic acid, the main metabolite of 5-HT.
iatrogenic	Induced by the doctor or treatment.

labyrinth	The inner ear, involved in hearing and balance.
latency	The interval between administering a drug and seeing a response.
ligand	A specific agent which binds to a receptor.
limbic system	Interconnected structures in the brain which are thought to be concerned with emotional and behavioural functions.
lipid soluble	Something which dissolves in fat; once a substance dissolves in fat it is removed from the body more slowly than substances which stay in the blood or enter other types of tissue.
LOS	Lower oesophageal sphincter.
mg	Milligram 10^{-3} of a gram (0.001 g).
µg (mcg)	Microgram 10^{-6} of a gram (0.000001 g).
neurotransmitter	A chemical which is released from a nerve ending to cross the small space between the nerve and the next cell (another nerve, a muscle, a blood vessel etc.) and has an effect on the receiving cell.
ng	Nanogram 10^{-9} of a gram (0.000000001 g).
NTS	Nucleus of the solitary tract.
nucleus	Central controlling structure of a cell. In neuroanatomical terms a nucleus is composed of cell bodies and is a co-ordinating structure within a nervous pathway, linking incoming and outgoing impulses.
parasympathetic	The part of the autonomic nervous system whose activity is classically associated with the state of the body after a meal (i.e. an increase in blood supply to the gut, and a decrease in blood supply to skin and muscles).
peptides	Molecules composed of a few amino acids. Larger chains of amino acids are oligopeptides, and above a certain size they are proteins.

peristalsis Regular waves of muscular contraction which give rise to a sequential squeezing of the gut to move its contents along.

pharmacokinetics The study of the absorption, distribution and elimination of a drug. Most of the subject involves a study of plasma levels.

placebo A 'dummy' pill or injection, containing no active ingredients. In clinical trials placebos are matched in appearance and dosage to the active drug. Consequently the patient, and often the nurse or doctor, do not know whether the patient is receiving active drug or is a control. If the patient alone is unaware of the nature of the treatment it is a single-blind trial; if the patient and the doctor are both unaware, it is a double-blind trial.

PMRT Progressive muscle relaxation training or therapy.

SSRI Selective serotonin reuptake inhibitor.

TBI Total body irradiation.

THC delta-9-tetrahydrocannabinol (the active ingredient in cannabis).

VAS Visual analogue scale.

VC Vomiting centre.

REFERENCES

Aapro, M.S. & Alberts, D.S. (1981) High-dose dexamethasone for prevention of cisplatin-induced vomiting. *Cancer Chemother Pharmacol*, **7**, 11–14.

Adriani, J., Summers, F.W. & Anthony, S.O. (1961) Is the prophylactic use of antiemetics in surgical patients justified? *JAMA*, **175**, 666–671.

Akwari, O.E. (1983) The gastrointestinal tract in chemotherapy induced emesis. A final common pathway. *Drugs*, **25**, (Suppl. 1) 18–34.

Alexander, G.D., Skupski, J.N. & Brown, E.M. (1984) The role of nitrous oxide in postoperative nausea and vomiting. *Anesth Analg*, **63**, 175.

Allan, S.G., Cornbleet, M.A., Warrington, P.S. *et al.* (1984) Dexamethasone and high dose metoclopramide: efficacy in controlling cisplatin induced nausea and vomiting. *Br Med J*, **289**, 878–879.

Altmaier, E.M., Ross, W.E. & Moore, K. (1982) A pilot investigation of the psychologic functioning of patients with anticipatory vomiting. *Cancer*, **49**, 201–204.

Andersen, R. & Krohg, K. (1976) Pain as a major cause of postoperative nausea. *Can Anaesth Soc J*, **23**, 366.

Andrews, P.L.R. (1992) Physiology of nausea and vomiting. *Br J Anaesth*, **69**, (Suppl. 1) 2S–19S.

Andrews, P.L.R., Bhandari, P., Garland, S. *et al.* (1990a) Does retching have a function?: an experimental study in the ferret. *Pharmacodyn Ther (Life Science Advances)*, **9**, 135–152.

Andrews, P.L.R., Davis, C.J., Bingham, S. *et al.* (1990b) The abdominal visceral innervation and the emetic reflex: pathways, pharmacology and plasticity. *Can J Physiol Pharmacol*, **68**, 141–168.

Andrews, P.L.R. & Davis, C.J. (1993) The mechanism of emesis induced by anti-cancer therapies. In *Emesis in Anti-cancer Therapy Mechanisms and Treatment.* (eds. P.L.R. Andrews and G.J. Sanger). Chapman & Hall, London.

Andrews, P.L.R. & Hawthorn, J. (1988) The neurophysiology of nausea and vomiting. *Baillière's Clinical Gastroenterology*, **2**, 141–168.

Andrews, P.L.R., Rapeport, W.G. & Sanger, G.J. (1989) Neuropharmacology of emesis induced by anti-cancer therapy. *TiPS*, **9**, 334–341.

Andrews, P. & Whitehead, S. (1900) Pregnancy sickness. *News in Physiological Sciences (NIPS)*, **5**, 5–10.

Andrykowski, M.A. & Gregg, M.E. (1992) The role of psychological variables in post-chemotherapy nausea: anxiety and expectation. *Psychosomatic Med*, **54**, 48–58.

Andrykowski, M.A., Redd, W.H. & Hatfield, A.K. (1985) Development of anticipatory nausea: a prospective analysis. *J Consulting Clin Psychol*, **53**, 447–454.

Assaf, R.A.E., Clarke, R.S.J., Dundee, J.W. & Samuel, I.O. (1974) Studies of drugs given before anaesthesia. XXIV: Metoclopramide with morphine and pethidine. *Br J Anaesth*, **46**, 514–519.

Bakowski, M.R. (1984) Advances in anti-emetic therapy. *Cancer Treatment Rev*, **11**, 237–256.

Barnett, K. (1972) A theoretical construct of the concepts of touch as they relate to nursing. *Nursing Res*, **21**, 102–110.

Barsoum, G., Perry, E.P. & Fraser, I.A. (1990) Postoperative nausea is relieved by acupressure. *J Roy Soc Med*, **83**, 86.

Bateman, D.N., Darling, W.M., Boys, R. & Rawlins, M.D. (1989) Extrapyramidal reactions to metoclopramide and prochlorperazine. *Q J Med*, **264**, 307–311.

Beattie, W.S., Lindblad, T., Buckley, D.N. & Forrest, J.B. (1991) The incidence of post-operative nausea and vomiting in women undergoing laparoscopy is influenced by the day of the menstrual cycle. *Can J Anaesth*, **38** 298–302.

Bellville, J.W., Bross, I.D.J. & Howland, W.S. (1960) Postoperative nausea and vomiting: IV. Factors related to postoperative nausea and vomiting. *Anesthesiology*, **21**, 186–193.

Benner, P. (1984) *From Novice to Expert Excellence and Power in Clinical Nursing Practice.* Addison-Wesley Publishing Co., Menlo Park, California.

Benrubi, G.I., Norvell, M., Nuss, R.C. & Robinson, H. (1985) The use of methylprednisolone and metoclopramide in control of emesis in patients receiving cisplatinum. *Gynecologic Oncology*, **21**, 306–313.

Benz, C., Gandara, D., Miller, B. *et al.* (1987) Chemoendocrine therapy with prolonged estrogen priming in advanced breast cancer: endocrine pharmacokinetics and toxicity. *Cancer Treat Rep*, **71**, 283–289.

Bermudez, J., Boyle, E.A., Miner, W.D. & Sanger, G.J. (1988) The anti-emetic potential of the 5-hydroxytryptamine receptor antagonist BRL43694. *Br J Cancer*, **58**, 644–650.

Bleiberg, H., Van Belle, S., Paridaens R. *et al.* (1992) Compassionate use of a 5-HT$_3$ receptor antagonist, tropisetron, in patients refractory to standard antiemetic treatment. *Drugs*, **43**, (Suppl. 3) 27–32.

Bodman, R.I., Morton, H.J.V. & Thomas, E.T. (1960) Vomiting by outpatients after nitrous oxide anaesthesia. *Br Med J*, **1**, 1372.

Boguslawski, M. (1980) Therapeutic touch: a facilitator of pain relief. *Topics in Cancer Nursing*, **2** (1) 27–37.

Bone, M.E., Wilkinson, D.J., Young, J.R. & Charlton, S. (1990) Ginger root – a new antiemetic. The effects of ginger root on postoperative nausea and vomiting after major gynaecological surgery. *Anaesthesia*, **45**, 669–671.

Bonica, J.J., Crepps, W., Monk, B. *et al.* (1958) Postoperative nausea retching and vomiting. *Anesthesiology*, **19**, 532–540.

Bonneterre, J. & Hecquet, B. (1993) Granisetron IV compared with ondansetron IV plus tablets in the prevention of nausea and vomiting induced by a moderately emetogenic chemotherapy regimen: a randomized crossover study. SB Symposium Antiemetic control: maximizing the benefits *Abstract Book*. ECCO 7.

Bradley, P.B., Engel, G., Fenuik, W. *et al.* (1986) Proposals for the classification and nomenclature of functional receptors for 5-hydroxytryptamine. *Neuropharmacol*, **25**, 563–576.

Bricourt, P. & McKenzie, J. (1984) Radiotherapy from the patient's viewpoint. In: *Radiation Therapy and Thanatology* (eds R. Torpie, L. Liegner & C. Chang). Springfield, Illinois, C. Charles Thomas.

Brock-Utne, J.G., Rubin, J., Welman, S. *et al.* (1978) The action of commonly used antiemetics on the lower oesophageal sphincter. *Br J Anaesth*, **26**, 295–298.

Bromage, P.R., Camporesi, E.M., Durant, P.A.C. & Neilsen, C.H. (1982) Nonrespiratory side effects of epidural morphine. *Anesth Analg*, **61**, 276–310.

Bruijn, K.M. (1992) Tropisetron. A review of clinical experience. *Drugs*, **43**, (Suppl. 3) 11–22.

Bruntsch, U. (1990) Enhanced efficacy by the addition of dexamethasone to ondansetron in cisplatin-induced emesis. *Zofran (ondansetron) Satellite Symposium. European Society for Medical Oncology*, Copenhagen, December 2. Copenhagen Falkoner Centre, Glaxo, 19–22.

Bruntsch, U., Drechsler, S., Hiller, E. *et al.* (1992) Prevention of chemotherapy-induced nausea and emesis in patients responding poorly to previous antiemetic therapy. *Drugs*, **43**, (Suppl. 3) 23–26.

Burish, T.G. & Carey, M.P. (1986) Conditioned aversive responses in cancer chemotherapy patients: theoretical and developmental analysis. *J Consulting Clin Psychol*, **54**, 593–600.

Burish, T.G., Carey, M.P., Krozely, M.G. & Greco, F.A. (1987) Conditioned side effects induced by cancer chemotherapy: prevention through behavioral treatment. *J Consulting Clin Psychol*, **55**, 42–48.

Burtles, R. & Peckett, B.W. (1957) Postoperative vomiting. *Br J Anaesth*, **29**, 114–123.

Byass, R. (1988) Soothing body and soul. *Nursing Times*, **84**, 24, 39–41.

Carey, M.P. & Burish, T.G. (1988) Etiology and treatment of the psychological side effects associated with cancer chemotherapy: a critical review and discussion. *Psychol Bull*, **104**, 307–325.

Carl. P.L., Cubeddu, L.X., Lindley, C. *et al.* (1989) Do humoral factors mediate cancer chemotherapy induced emesis? *Drug Metab Rev*, **21**, 319–333.

Carrie, L.E.S. & Simpson, P.J. (1988) *Understanding Anaesthesia*. William Heinemann, London.

Cassileth, A., Lusk, E.J., Torri, S., *et al.* (1983) Antiemetic efficacy of dexamethasone therapy in patients receiving cancer chemotherapy. *Arch Intern Med*, **143**, 1347–1349.

Chevallier, B. (1990) Efficacy and safety of granisetron compared with high-dose metoclopramide plus dexamethasone in patients receiving high-dose cisplatin in a single-blind study. *Eur J Cancer*, **26**, (Suppl 1) S33–S36.

Clarke, R.S.J. (1984) Nausea and vomiting. *Br J Anaesth*, **56**, 19.

Clarke, R.S.J. (1991) Post-operative gastrointestinal complications. *Current Anaes Crit Care*, **2**, 20–24.

Coates, A., Abraham, S., Kaye, S.B. *et al.* (1983) On the receiving end – patient perception of the side-effects of cancer chemotherapy. *Eur J Cancer Clin Oncol*, **19**, 203–208.

Cohen, M.M., Cameron, C.B. & Duncan, P.G. (1990) Pediatric anesthesia morbidity and mortality in the postoperative period. *Anesth Analg*, **70**, 160–167.

Comroe, J.H. & Dripps, R.D. (1948) Reaction to morphine in ambulatory and bed patients. *Surg Gynecol Obstet*, **87**, 221.

Cookson, R.F. (1986) Mechanisms and treatment of post-operative nausea and vomiting. In: *Nausea and Vomiting: Mechanisms and Treatment* (eds C.J. Davis, G.V. Lake-Bakaar, D.G. Grahame-Smith), pp. 130–150, Springer-Verlag.

Coons, H.L., Leventhal, H., Nerenz, D.R. *et al.* (1987) Anticipatory nausea and emotional distress in patients receiving cisplatin-based chemotherapy. *Oncology Nursing Forum*, **14**, 31.

Copley Cobb, S. (1984) Teaching relaxation to cancer patients. *Cancer Nursing*, **7**, 157–161.

Costall, B., Domeney, A.M., Gunning, S.J., Naylor, R.J., Tattersall, F.D. & Tyers, M.B. (1987) GR38032F: a potent and novel inhibitor of cis-platin-induced emesis in the ferret. *Br J Pharmacol*, **90**, 90P.

Cotanch, P.H. (1983) Relaxation training for control of nausea and vomiting in patients receiving chemotherapy. *Cancer Nursing*, **6**(4), 277–283.

Cousins, M.J. & Mather, L.E. (1984) Intrathecal and epidural adminis-tration of opioids. *Anesthesiology*, **61**, 276–310.

Creytens, G. (1984) Effect of the non-antidopaminergic drug cisapride on postprandial nausea. *Current Ther Res*, **36**, 1063–1070.

Crocker, J.S. & Vandam, L.D. (1959) Concerning nausea and vomiting during spinal anaesthesia. *Anesthesiology*, **20**, 589–592.

Cronin, M., Redfern, P.A. & Utting, J.E. (1973) Psychometry and post-operative complaints in surgical patients. *Br J Anaesth*, **45**, 879–886.

Cubeddu, L.X. (1993) The role of serotonin in chemotherapy-induced emesis in cancer patients. In: *Anti-emetic Therapy: Current Status and Future Prospects*, (eds Rubio E. Diaz & M. Martin). Glaxo, pp. 41–45.

Cubeddu, L.X., Hoffman, I.S., Fuenmayor, N.T. & Finn, A.F. (1990) Efficacy of ondansetron (GR 38032F) and the role of serotonin in cisplatin-induced nausea and vomiting. *N Eng J Med*, **322**, 810–816.

Cull, A. (1993) Psychological effects of anti-cancer therapy. In: *Emesis in Anti-cancer Therapy. Mechanisms and Treatment* (eds P.L.R. Andrews and G.J. Sanger), Chapman & Hall, London.

Cunningham, D., Bradley, C.J., Forrest, G.J. *et al.* (1988) A randomized trial of oral nabilone and prochlorperazine compared to intravenous metoclopramide and dexamethasone in the treatment of nausea and vomiting induced by chemotherapy regimens containing cisplatin or cisplatin analogues. *Eur J Cancer Clin Oncol*, **24**, 685–689.

Cunningham, D.C., Forrest, G.J., Soukop, M. *et al.* (1985a) Nabilone and prochloperazine: a useful combination for emesis induced by cytotoxic drugs. *Br Med J*, **291**, 864–865.

Cunningham, D.C., Soukop, M., Gilchrist, N.L. *et al.* (1985b) Randomized trial of intravenous high dose metoclopramide and intramuscular chlorpromazine in controlling nausea and vomiting induced by cytotoxic drugs. *Br Med J*, **290**, 604–605.

D'Acquisto, R.W., Tyson, L.B. & Gralla, R.J. (1986) The influence of a chronic high alcohol intake on chemotherapy-induced nausea and vomiting. *Proc Am Soc Clin Oncol*, **5**, 257.

Datta, S., Alper, M.H., Ostheimer, G.W. & Weiss, J.B. (1982) Method of ephedrine administration and nausea and hypotension during spinal anaesthesia for cesarean section. *Anesthesiology*, **56**, 68.

Davidson, H.I.M. & Pilot, M-A. (1993) Changes in gastro-intestinal motility associated with vomiting and nausea. In: *Emesis in Anticancer Therapy: Mechanisms and Treatment* (eds P.L.R. Andrews and G.J. Sanger), Chapman & Hall, London.

Davis, C.J., Harding, R.K., Leslie, R.A. & Andrews, P.L.R. (1986) The organisation of vomiting as a protective reflex: A commentary on the first day's discussions. In: *Nausea and Vomiting: Mechanisms and Treatment*, (eds C.J. Davis, G.V. Lake-Bakaar & D.G. Grahame-Smith) pp. 65–75, Springer Verlag.

Davis, I., Moore, J.R.M. & Lahiri, S.K. (1979) Nitrous oxide and the middle ear. *Anaesthesia*, **34**, 147–151.

Davson, H., Welch, K. & Segal, M.B. (1987) Physiology and pathophysiology of the cerebrospinal fluid. In: *The Cerebrospinal Fluid Pressure*. Chap 14, pp. 731–782. Churchill Livingstone, Edinburgh.

De Mulder, P., Seyenaeve, C., Vermorken, J. *et al.* (1990) Ondansetron compared with high-dose metoclopramide in the prophylaxis of acute and delayed cisplatin-induced nausea and vomiting – a multicentre randomised, double-blind, crossover study. *Annals Int Med*, **113**, 834–840.

Del Favero, A., Roila, F., Basurto, C. *et al.* (1990) Assessment of nausea. *Eur J Clin Pharmacol*, **38**, 115–120.

Del Favero, A., Tonato, M. & Roila, F. (1992) Issues in the measurement of nausea. *Br J Cancer*, **66**, (Suppl. XIX) S69–S71.

Dilly, S.G. (1993) A double-blind cross-over study to compare the efficacy and safety of granisetron and ondansetron in the prophylaxis of nausea and vomiting induced by 5-day fractionated chemotherapy. SB Symposium Antiemetic Control: Maximizing the Benefits Abstract Book. ECCO 7.

DiSilva, K.L., Muller, P.J. & Pearce, J. (1973) Acute drug-induced extrapyramidal syndromes. *Practitioner*, **211**, 316–320.

Dogliotti, L., Antonacci, R.A., Paze, E. *et al.* (1992) Three years' experience with tropisetron in the control of nausea and vomiting in cisplatin-treated patients. *Drugs,* **43**, (Suppl. 3) 6–10.

Dolgin, M.J., Katz, E.R., McGinty, K. & Siegel, S.E. (1985) Anticipatory nausea and vomiting in pediatric patients. *Pediatrics,* **75**, 547–552.

D'Olimpio, J.T., Camacho, F.J., Chandra, P. *et al.* (1984) Anti-emetic treatment of patients receiving cisplatin based chemotherapy with high dose dexamethasone versus placebo: a randomized double-blind controlled clinical trial. *ASCO,* **3**, 95.

Donovan, M.I. (1980) Relaxation with guided imagery: a useful technique. *Cancer Nursing,* **3**, 27–32.

Donovitz, G.S., O'Quinn, A.G. & Smith, M.L. (1984) Antiemetic efficacy of high-dose corticosteroids and droperidol in cisplatin-induced emesis: a controlled trial with droperidol and metoclopramide. *Gynaecologic Oncol,* **18**, 320–325.

D'Souza, D.P., Reyntjens, A. & Thomas, R.D. (1980) Domperidone in the prevention of nausea and vomiting induced by antineoplastic agents: a threefold evaluation. *Cur Ther Res,* **27**, 384–390.

Dundee, J.W. (1988) Acupuncture/acupressure as an antiemetic: studies of its use in postoperative vomiting, cancer chemotherapy and sickness of early pregnancy. *Complementary Med Res,* **3**, 1–14.

Dundee, J.W., Assaf, R.A.E, Loan, W.B. & Morrison, J.D. (1975) A comparison of the efficacy of cyclizine and perphenazine in reducing the emetic effects of morphine and pethidine. *Br J Clin Pharm,* **2**, 81–85.

Dundee, J.W., Ghaly, R.G., Fitzpatrick, K.T.J. *et al.* (1989) Acupuncture prophylaxis of cancer chemotherapy-induced sickness. *J Roy Soc Med,* **82**, 268–271.

Dundee, J.W., Kirwan, M.J. & Clarke, R.S.J. (1965) Anaesthesia and premedication as factors in post-operative vomiting. *Acta Anaesthesiol Scand,* **9**, 223.

Dundee, J.W., Nicholl, R.M. & Moore, J. (1962) Studies of drugs given before anaesthesia. III: A method for the studying of their effects on postoperative vomiting and nausea. *Br J Anaesth,* **34**, 527.

Dundee, J.W. & Yang, J. (1990) Prolongation of the antiemetic action of P6 acupuncture by acupressure in patients having cancer chemotherapy. *J Roy Soc Med,* **83**, 360–362.

Du Pen, S., Scuderi, P., Wetchler, B. *et al.* (1992) Ondanstron in the treatment of postoperative nausea and vomiting in ambulatory outpatients: a dose-comparative, stratified, multicentre study. *Eur J Anaesthesiol,* **9**, (Suppl. 6) 55–62.

Ellis, F.R. & Spence, A.A. (1970) Clinical trials of metoclopramide as an antiemetic in anaesthesia. *Anaesthesia,* **25**, 368–371.

Enck, R.E. (1977) Mallory-Weiss lesion following cancer chemotherapy. *Lancet,* Oct 29: 927–928.

Fetting, J.H., Gruchow, L.B., Fuerstein, M.F. *et al.* (1982) The course of nausea and vomiting after high-dose cyclophosphamide. *Cancer Treat Rep*, **66**, 1487–1493.

Finlay, I. (1991) Rational use of antiemetics in the terminally ill. *Postgrad Update*, 1 December, 876–880.

Forrest, J.B., Cahalan, M.K., Rehder, K. *et al.* (1990) Multicentre study of general anaesthesia II. Results. *Anesthesiology*, **72**, 262–268.

Fozard, J.R. & Mobarok-Ali, A.T.M. (1978) Blockade of neuronal tryptamine receptors by metoclopramide. *Eur J Pharmacol*, **49**, 109–112.

Frazer, N.M., Felgate, L. Keery, R.J. & Keene, O.N. (1991) Tolerability of intravenous dosing of ondansetron 16mg. *Br J Clin Pharm*, **32**, 235P.

Friesen, R.H. & Lockhart, C.H. (1992) Oral transmucosal fentanyl citrate for preanesthetic medication of pediatric day surgery patients with and without droperidol as a prophylactic anti-emetic. *Anesthesiology*, **76**, 46–51.

Gaddum, J.H. & Picarelli, Z.P. (1957) Two kinds of tryptamine receptor. *Br J Pharmacol*, **12**, 323–328.

Gaskey, N.J., Pournaras, L., Ferrerio, L. & Seecof, J. (1986) Use of fentanyl markedly increases nausea and vomiting in gynecological short stay patients. *J Assoc Nurs Anes*, **54**, 309–311.

Gillman, M.A. (1985) Nitrous oxide and its opioid properties. *Can Anaesth Soc J*, **32**, 315.

Grahn, G. (1988) Developing an education and support programme for cancer patients and their family members. In: *Cancer Nursing – A Revolution in Care*, pp. 53–56, (ed. A.P. Pritchard). Macmillan, London.

Grahn, G. & Johnson, J. (1990) Learning to cope and living with cancer. Learning-needs assessment in cancer patient education. *Scand J Can Science*, **4**, 4.

Gralla, R.J. (1983) Metroclopramide. *Drugs*, **25**, (Suppl. 1) 63–73.

Gralla, R.J., Itri, L.M., Pisko, S.E. *et al.* (1981) Antiemetic efficacy of high-dose metoclopramide: randomized trials with placebo and prochlorperazine in patients with chemotherapy-induced nausea and vomiting. *New Eng J Med*, **3055**, 905–909.

Gralla, R.J., Tyson, L.B., Kris, M.G. & Clark, R.A. (1987) The management of chemotherapy-induced nausea and vomiting. *Med Clin North America*, **71**(2), 289–301.

Grunberg, S.M., Gala, K.V. & Lampenfeld, M. (1984) Comparison of the antiemetic effect of high-dose intravenous metoclopramide and high-dose intravenous haloperidol in a randomized double-blind cross-over study. *Cancer*, **60**(2), 2816–2811.

Gunwardene, R.D. & White, D.C. (1988) Propofol and emesis. *Anaesthesia*, **43**, (Suppl.) 65–67.

Gylys, J.A., Doran, K.M. & Buyniski, J.P. (1979) Antagonism of cisplatin induced emesis in the dog. *Res. Comm Chem Pathol Pharmacol*, **23**, 61–68.

Hackett, G.H., Harris, M.N.E., Plantevin, H.M., Pringle, D.B. &

Avery, A.J. (1982) Anaesthesia for outpatient termination of pregnancy. *Br J Anaesth*, **54**, 865–879.

Hainsworth, J., Harvey, W., Pendergrass, K. *et al.* (1991) A single-blind comparison of intravenous ondansetron, a selective serotonin antagonist, with intravenous metoclopramide in the prevention of nausea and vomiting associated with high-dose cisplatin chemotherapy. *J Clin Oncol*, **9**, 721–728.

Handley, A.J. (1967) Metoclopramide in the prevention of postoperative nausea and vomiting. *Br J Clin Pract*, **21**, 460.

Haumann, J. & Foster, P. (1963) The antiemetic effect of halothane. *Br J Anaesth*, **35**, 114–117.

Hawthorn, J. & Cunningham, D. (1990) Dexamethasone can potentiate the anti-emetic action of a 5-HT$_3$ receptor antagonist on cyclophosphamide-induced vomiting in the ferret. *Br J Cancer*, **61**, 56–60.

Hawthorn, J., Ostler, K.J. & Andrews, P.L.R. (1988) The role of the abdominal visceral innervation and 5-HT-M receptors in vomiting induced by the cytotoxic drugs cyclophosphamide and cisplatin in the ferret. *Q J Exp Physiol*, **73**, 7–21.

Headley, J.A. (1987) The influence of administration time on chemotherapy-induced nausea and vomiting. *Oncol Nurs Forum*, **14**(6), 43–47.

Hogan, C.M. (1990) Advances in the management of nausea and vomiting. *Nurs Clin N Amer*, **25**, 475–497.

Holli, K. (1993) Ineffectiveness of relaxation on vomiting induced by cancer chemotherapy. *Eur J Cancer*, **29A**, 1915–1916.

Hovorka, J., Korttila, K. & Erkola, O. (1989) Nitrous oxide does not increase nausea and vomiting following gynaecological laparoscopy. *Can J Anaesth*, **36**, 145–148.

Hovorka, J., Korttila, K. & Erkola, O. (1990) The experience of the person ventilating the lungs does influence postoperative nausea and vomiting. *Acta Anaesthes Scand*, **34**, 203–205.

Howarth, F.H., Cockel, R., Roper, B.W. & Hawkins, C.F. (1969) The effect of metoclopramide upon gastric motility and its value in barium progress meals. *Clin Radiology*, **20**, 294–300.

Humphrey, P.P.A., Hartig, P. & Hoyer, D. (1993) A proposed new nomenclature for 5-HT receptors. *TiPS*, **14**, 233–236.

Ingle, R.J., Burish, T.G. & Wallston, K.A. (1984) Conditionability of cancer chemotherapy patients. *Oncol Nurs Forum*, **11**, 97–102.

Ireland, J. & Tyers, M.B. (1987) Pharmacological characterization of 5-hydroxytryptamine-induced depolarization of the rat isolated vagus nerve. *Br J Pharmacol*, **90**, 229–238.

Italian Group for Antiemetic Research (1992) Ondansetron + dexamethasone vs metoclopramide + dexamethasone + diphenhydramine in prevention of cisplatin-induced emesis. *Lancet*, **340**, 96–99.

Iwamoto, K. & Schwartz, H. (1978) Antiemetic effect of droperidol after ophthalmic surgery. *Arch Ophthalmol*, **96**, 1378–1379.

Jacobson, P.B., Andrykowski, M.A., Redd, W.H. *et al.* (1988) Non pharmacologic factors in the development of post-treatment nausea with adjuvant chemotherapy for breast cancer. *Cancer*, **61**, 379–385.

Jantunen, I.T. Muhonen, T.T., Kataja, V.V., Flander, M.K. & Terenhovi, L. (1993) 5-HT$_3$ receptor antagonists in the prophylaxis of acute vomiting induced by moderately emetogenic chemotherapy – a randomised study. *Eur J Cancer*, **29A**, 1669–1672.

Jarnfelt-Samsioe, A. (1987) Nausea and vomiting in pregnancy: a review. *Obstet Gynaecol Survey*, **41**, 422–427.

Johnson, J., Nail, L., Lauver, D. *et al.* (1988) Reducing the negative impact of radiation therapy on functional status. *Cancer*, **61**, 46–51.

Johnson, J.E., Rice, V.H., Fuller, S.S. & Endress, M.P. (1978) Sensory information instructions in coping strategy and recovery from surgery. *Res Nurs Health*, **1**, 4–17.

Jones, A.L. Cunningham, D., Soukop, M. *et al.* (1991) Comparison of dexamethasone and ondansetron in the prophylaxis of emesis induced by moderately emetogenic chemotherapy. *Lancet*, **338**, 483–487.

Jordan, L.N. (1989) Effects of fluid manipulation on the incidence of vomiting during outpatient cisplatin infusion. *Oncol Nurs Forum*, **16**, 213–218.

Kamath, B., Curran, J., Hawkey, C. *et al.* (1990) Anaesthesia, movement and emesis. *Br J Anaesth*, **64**, 728–730.

Kilpatrick, G.J., Jones, B.J. & Tyers, M.B. (1988) The distribution of specific binding of the 5-HT$_3$ receptor ligand [^{3}H] GR65630 in rat brain using quantitative autoradiography. *Neurosci Letts*, **94**, 156–160.

King, M.J., Milazkiewicz, R., Carli, F. & Deacock, A.R. (1988) Influence of neostigmine on post-operative vomiting. *Br J Anaesth*, **61**, 403–406.

Knapp, M.R. & Beecher, H.K. (1956) Postanaesthetic nausea, vomiting and retching. *JAMA*, **160**, 376–385.

Korttila, K., Hovorka, J. & Erkola, O. (1987) Nitrous oxide does not increase the incidence of nausea and vomiting after isoflurane anesthesia. *Anesth Analg*, **66**, 761–765.

Korttila, K., Kauste, A. & Auvinen, J. (1979) Comparison of domperidone, droperidol, and metoclopramide in the prevention and treatment of nausea and vomiting after balanced general anaesthesia. *Anesth Analg*, **58**, 396–400.

Kovac, A., McKenzie, R., O'Connor, T. *et al.* (1992) Prophylactic intravenous ondansetron in female outpatients undergoing gynaecological surgery: a multicentre dose-comparison study. *Eur J Anaesthsiol*, **9**, (Suppl. 6) 37–48.

Krieger, D. (1975) Therapeutic touch: the imprimatur of nursing. *Am J Nursing*, **75**, 784–787.

Kris, M.G., Gralla, R.J., Clark, R.A. *et al.* (1985a) Incidence, course, and severity of delayed nausea and vomiting following the administration of high-dose cisplatin. *J Clin Oncol*, **3**, 1379–1384.

Kris, M.G., Gralla, R.J., Clark, R.A. *et al.* (1987) Antiemetic control and prevention of side effects of anti-cancer therapy with lorazepam or diphenhydramine when used in combination with metoclopramide plus dexamethasone. *Cancer*, **60**, 2816–2822.

Kris, M.G., Gralla, R.J., Tyson, L.B. *et al.* (1985b) Improved control of cisplatin-induced emesis with high-dose metoclopramide and with combinations of metoclopramide, dexamethasone, and diphenhydramine. *Cancer*, **55**, 527–534.

Kris, M.G., Tyson, L.B. & Gralla, R.J. (1983) Extrapyramidal reactions with high-dose metoclopramide. *New Eng J Med*, **309**, 433.

Kvisselgaard, N. (1958) Chlorpromazine and cyclizine in the prevention of postoperative nausea and vomiting. *Acta Anaesthesiol Scand*, **2**, 153.

Lang, I.M. (1990) Digestive tract motor correlates of nausea and vomiting. *Can J Physiol Pharmacol*, **68**, 242–253.

Larsson, S., Asgeirsson, B. & Magnusson, J. (1992) Propofol-fentanyl anaesthesia compared to thiopental-halothane with special reference to recovery and vomiting after pediatric strabismus surgery. *Acta Anaesthesiol Scand*, **36**, 182–186.

Laszlo, J., Clarke, R.A., Hanson, D.C. *et al.* (1985) Lorazepam in cancer patients treated with cisplatin: a drug having antiemetic, amnesic, and anxiolytic effects. *J Clin Oncol*, **3**, 864–869.

Lawson, M., Kern, F. & Everson, G.T. (1985) Gastrointestinal transit time in human pregnancy: prolongation in the second and third trimesters followed by post partum normalization. *Gastroenterology*, **89**, 966–999.

Lee, K.Y., Park, H.J. & Chey, W.Y. (1985) Studies of mechanisms of retching and vomiting in dogs. *Dig Dis Sci*, **30**, 22–28.

Lerman, J. (1992) Surgical and patient factors involved in postoperative nausea and vomiting. *Br J Anaesth*, **69**, (Suppl. 1) 24S–32S.

Lerman, J., Eustis, S. & Smith, D.R. (1986) Effect of droperidol pretreatment on postanesthetic vomiting in children undergoing strabismus surgery. *Anesthesiology*, **65**, 322–325.

Leslie, R.A. (1985) Neuroactive substances in the dorsal vagal complex of the medulla oblongata: nucleus of the solitary tract, area postrema and dorsal nucleus of the vagus. *Neurochem Int*, **7**, 191–211.

Leslie, R.A. & Gwyn, D.G. (1984) Neuronal connections of the area postrema. *Fed Proc*, **43**, 2941–2943.

Leslie, R.A., Reynolds, D.J.M., Andrews, P.L.R. *et al.* (1990) Evidence for presynaptic 5-hydroxytryptamine$_3$ recognition sites on vagal afferent terminals in the brainstem of the ferret. *Neuroscience* **38**, 667–673.

Lessin, J.B., Azad, S.S., Rosenblum, F., Bartkowski, R.R. & Marr, A. (1991) Does antiemetic prophylaxis with ondansetron prolong recovery time? *Anesth Analg.*, **72** (2S), S162.

Lin, D.M., Furst, S.R. & Rodarte, A. (1992) A double-blind comparison of metoclopramide and droperidol for prevention of emesis following strabismus surgery. *Anesthesiology*, **76**, 357–361.

Linblad, T., Beattie, W.S., Forrest, J.B. & Buckley, D.N. (1990) Loss of antiemetic effect of droperidol in menstruating women. *Can J. Anaesth*, **37**, S139.

Lind, B.C. & Breivik, H. (1970) Metoclopramide and perphenazine in the prevention of postoperative nausea and vomiting. *Br J Anaesth*, **42**, 614–617.

Lindley, C.M., Bernard, S. & Fields, S.F. (1989) Incidence and duration of chemotherapy-induced nausea and vomiting in the outpatient oncology population. *J Clin Oncol*, **7**, 1142–1149.

Liotti, V.J. & Clark, C. (1974) Carbidopa attenuation of L-Dopa emesis in dogs: evidence for a cerebral site of action outside the blood brain barrier. *Eur J Pharmacol*, **25**, 322–325.

Loan, W.B., Dundee, J.W. & Clarke, R.S.J. (1966) Studies of drugs given before anaesthesia XII. A comparison of papaveretum and morphine. *Br J Anaesth*, **38**, 891–900.

Loeser, E.A., Bennet, G., Stanley, T.H. & Machin, R. (1979) Comparison of droperidol, haloperidol and prochlorperazine as postoperative antiemetics. *Can Anaesth Soc J*, **26**, 125–127.

Logue, J.P., Magee, B., Hunter, R.D. & Murdoch, R.D. (1991) The antiemetic of granisetron in lower hemibody radiotherapy. *Clin Oncol*, **3**, 247–249.

Lonie, D.S. & Harper, N.J.N. (1986) Nitrous oxide anaesthesia and vomiting. *Anaesthesia*, **41**, 703–707.

Loper, K.A., Ready, L.B. & Dorman, B.H. (1989) Prophylactic trans-dermal scopolamine patches reduce nausea in postoperative patients receiving epidural morphine. *Anesth Analg*, **68**, 144–146.

McAteer, P.M., Carter, J.A., Cooper, G.M. & Prys-Roberts, C. (1986) Comparison of isoflurane and halothane in outpatient paediatric dental anaesthesia. *Br J Anaesth*, **58**, 390–393.

McCarthy, L.E. & Borison, H.L. (1974) Respiratory mechanics of vomiting in decerebrate cats. *Am J Physiol*, **226**, 738–743.

McCaul, K.D. & Malott, J.M. (1984) Distraction and coping with pain. *Psych Bull*, **95**, 518–533.

McDermed, J.E. (1983) A randomized, cross-over comparison of the effectiveness of intravenous (IV) metoclopramide (MCP) and IV dexamethasone (DXM) as antiemetic prevention in cancer chemotherapy (CT). *ASCO*, **2**, 88.

McKenzie, R., Wadhwa, R.K., Lim, N.T. *et al.* (1981) Antiemetic effectiveness of intramuscular hydroxyzine compared with intramuscular droperidol. *Anesth Analg*, **60**, 783–788.

Marschner, N. (1991) Anti-emetic control with ondansetron in the chemotherapy of breast cancer: a review. *Eur J Cancer*, **27**, (Suppl. 1) S15–S17.

Martin, M. & Diaz-Rubio, E. (1990) Emesis during past pregnancy: A new prognostic factor in chemotherapy-induced emesis. *Annals Oncol*, **1**, 152–153.

Marty, M. (1990) A comparative study of the use of granisetron, a selective 5-HT$_3$ receptor antagonist, versus a standard antiemetic regimen of chlorpromazine plus dexamthasone in the treatment of cytostatic-induced emesis. *Eur J Cancer*, **26**, (Suppl. 1) S33–SS36.

Marty, M., Pouillart, P., Scholl, S. *et al.* (1990) Comparison of the 5-hydroxytryptamine-3 (serotonin) antagonist ondansetron (GR38032F) with high-dose metoclopramide in the control of cis-platin-induced emesis. *New Eng J Med*, **322**, 816–821.

Melnick, B.M., Chalasani, J. & Uy, N.T.L. (1984) Comparison of enflurane, isoflurane and continuous fentanyl infusion for outpatient anesthesia. *Anesthesiol Rev*, **11**, 36–39.

Melnick, B.M. & Johnson, L.S. (1987) Effect of eliminating nitrous oxide in outpatient anesthesia. *Anesthesiology*, **67**, 982–984.

Mercadante, S., Spoldi, E., Caraceni, A., Maddaloni, S. & Simonetti, M.T. (1993) Orectide in relieving gastrointestinal symptoms due to bowel obstruction. *Pall Med*, **7**, 295–299.

Meyer, B.R., Lewin, M. & Dreyer, D.E. (1984) Optimizing metoclopra-mide control of cisplatin-induced emesis. *N Eng J Med*, **100**, 393–395.

Miner, W.D. & Sanger, G.J. (1986) Inhibition of cisplatin-induced vomiting by selective 5-hydroxytryptamine M-receptor antagonism. *Br J Pharmacol*, **88**, 497–499.

Mori, M.N., Amino, H., Tamaki, K. *et al.* (1988) Morning sickness and thyroid function in normal pregnancy. *Obstet Gynaecol*, **72**, 355–359.

Morrison, J.D., Hill, G.B. & Dundee, J.W. (1968) Studies of drugs given before anaesthesia. XV. Evaluation of the method of study after 10 000 observations. *Br J Anaesth*, **40**, 890.

Morrow, G.R. (1984a) The assessment of nausea and vomiting. *Cancer*, **53**, (Suppl. 1) 2267–2280.

Morrow, G.R. (1984b) Susceptibility to motion sickness and the development of anticipatory nausea and vomiting in cancer patients undergoing chemotherapy and radiotherapy. *Cancer Treatment Rep*, **68**, 1177–1178.

Morrow, G.R. (1985) The effect of a susceptibility to motion sickness on the side effects of cancer chemotherapy. *Cancer*, **55**, 2766–2770.

Morrow, G.R. (1992) Behavioural factors influencing the development and expression of chemotherapy induced side effects. *Br J Cancer*, **66**, (Suppl. XIX) S54–S61.

Morrow, G.R. & Morrell, C. (1982) Behavioral treatment for the antici-patory nausea and vomiting induced by cancer chemotherapy. *New Eng J Med*, **307**, 1476–1480.

Muir, J.J., Warner, M.A., Offort, K.P., *et al.* (1987) Role of nitrous oxide and other factors in postoperative nausea and vomiting: a rando-mized and blinded prospective study. *Anesthesiology*, **66**, 513–518.

Nerenz, D.R., Leventhal, H., Easterling, D.V. & Love, R.R. (1986)

Anxiety and drug taste as predictors of anticipatory nausea in cancer chemotherapy. *J Clin Oncol*, **4**, 224–233.

Nesse, R.M., Carli, T., Curtis, G.C. *et al.* (1980) Pre-treatment nausea in cancer chemotherapy: a conditioned response? *Psychosom Med*, **42**, 43–46.

Nolan, E.M. (1985) Nausea, vomiting and dehydration. In: *Signs and Symptoms in Nursing Interpretation and Management.* (eds Margaret Jacobs and Wilma Geels). Lippencott and Co., Philadelphia.

Norman, D.K. & Herzog, D.B. (1986) A three-year outcome study of normal-weight bulimia: assessment of psychological functioning and eating attitudes. *Psychiatry Res*, **19**, 199–205.

Olver, I.N., Webster, L.K., Bishop, J.S. *et al.* (1989) A dose finding study of prochlorperazine as an anti-emetic for cancer chemotherapy. *Eur J Cancer Clin Oncol*, **25**, 1457–1461.

Orr, L.E., McKernan, J.F. & Bloome, B. (1980) Antiemetic effect of tetrahydrocannabinol compared with placebo and prochlorperazine in chemotherapy-associated nausea and emesis. *Arch Int Med*, **140**, 1431–1433.

Palazzo, M.G.A. & Strunin, L. (1984a) Anaesthesia and emesis. I: etiology. *Can Anaesth Soc J*, **31**, 178–187.

Palazzo, M.G.A. & Strunin, L. (1984b) Anaesthesia and emesis. II: Prevention and management. *Can Anaesth Soc J*, **31**, 407–415.

Parkhouse, J., Henrie, J.R., Duncan, G.M. & Rome, H.P. (1960) Nitrous oxide analgesia in relation to mental performance. *J Pharmacol Ther*, **128**, 44–54.

Parkhouse, J. (1963) The cure for postoperative vomiting. *Br J Anaesth*, **35**, 189.

Patton, C.N., Moon, M.R. & Dannemiller, F.J. (1974) The prophylactic antiemetic effect of droperidol. *Anesth Analg*, **53**, 361.

Pinkerton, C.R., Williams, D., Wooten, C., Meller, S.T. & McElwain, T.J. (1990) 5-HT$_3$ antagonist ondansetron – an effective outpatient antiemetic in cancer treatment. *Arch Dis Childhood*, **65**, 822–825.

Pratt, G.D., Bowery, N.G., Kilpatrick, G.J. *et al.* (1990) Consensus meeting agrees distribution of 5-HT$_3$ receptors in mammalian hindbrain. *TiPS*, **11**, 135–137.

Prentice, H.G. (1992) Granisetron in the prevention of radiotherapy-induced emesis. *Satellite Symposium to XVIIth Congress of ESMO.* Lyon, France.

Priestman, T. (1988) Radiation-induced emesis. *Clincian*, **6**(3), 40–43.

Priestman, T.J., Roberts, J.T., Lucraft, H., *et al.* (1990) Results of a randomized, double-blind comparative study of ondansetron and metoclopramide in the prevention of nausea and vomiting following high-dose upper abdominal irradiation. *Clin Oncol*, **2**, 71–75.

Pritchard, A.P. & Mallett, J. (eds) (1992) *The Royal Marsden Hospital Manual of Clinical Nursing Procedures.* Chapter 33, pp. 364–389. 3rd Edn, Blackwell Scientific Publications, Oxford.

Pritchard, A.P. & Speechley, V.D. (1990) What do nurses know about emesis? *International Cancer Nursing News*, **1**, 6–8.

Purkis, I.E. (1964), Factors that influence postoperative vomiting. *Can Anaesth Soc J*, **11**, 335–353.

Raftery, S. & Sherry, A. (1992) Total intravenous anaesthesia with propofol and alfentanil protects against postoperative nausea and vomiting. *Can J Anaesth*, **39**, 37–40.

Ratra, C.K., Badola, R.P. & Bhargava, K.P. (1972) A study of factors concerned in emesis during spinal anaesthesia. *Br J Anaesth*, **44**, 1208.

Reason, J.T. (1970) Motion sickness: a special case of sensory rearrangement. *Adv Sci*, **26**, 386–393.

Redd, W.H., Andresen, G.V. & Minagawa, R.Y. (1982) Hypnotic control of anticipatory emesis in patients receiving cancer chemotherapy. *J Consulting Clin Psychol*, **50**, 14–19.

Redd, W.H., Dadds, M.R., Futterman, A.D., Taylor, K.L. & Bovbjerg, D.H. (1993) Nausea induced by mental images of chemotherapy. *Cancer*, **72**, 629–636.

Regnard, C. & Comiskey, M. (1992) Nausea and vomiting in advanced cancer – flow diagram. *Pall Med*, **6**, 146–151.

Reynolds, D.J.M., Andrews, P.L.R., Leslie, R.A., *et al.* (1989) Bilateral abdominal vagotomy abolishes binding of ^{3}H BRL 43694 in ferret dorsovagal complex. *Br J Pharmacol*, **98** 692P.

Reynolds, D.J.M., Barber, N.A., Grahame-Smith, D.G. & Leslie, R.A. (1991) Cisplatin-evoked induction of c-fos protein in the brainstem of the ferret: the effect of cervical vagotomy and the anti-emetic 5-HT$_3$ receptor antagonist granisetron (BRL 43694). *Brain Res*, **565**, 231–236.

Reyntjens, A. (1979) Domperidone as an anti-emetic: summary of research reports. *Postgrad Med J*, **55**, (Suppl. 1) 50–54.

Rhodes, V.A., Watson, P.M. & Johnson, M.H. (1984) Development of reliable and valid measures of nausea and vomiting. *Cancer Nurs*, **7**(1), 33–41.

Rhodes, V.A., Watson, P.M. & Johnson, M.H. (1986) Association of chemotherapy related nausea and vomiting with pretreatment and posttreatment anxiety. *Oncol Nurs Forum*, **13**, 41.

Rich, W.M., Abdulhayoglu, G. & DiSaia, P.J. (1980) Methylprednisolone as an antiemetic during cancer chemotherapy – a pilot study. *Gynecologic Oncology*, **9**, 193–198.

Riding, J.E. (1960) Postoperative vomiting. *Proc Roy Soc Med*, **53**, 671–677.

Riding, J.E. (1975) Minor complications of general anaesthesia. *Br J Anaesth*, **47**, 91.

Rising, S., Dodgson, M.S. & Steen, P.A. (1985) Isoflurane *v.* fentanyl for outpatient laparoscopy. *Acta Anaesthesiol Scand*, **29**, 251–255.

Rita, L., Goodarzi, M. & Seleny, F. (1981) Effect of low dose droperidol on postoperative vomiting in children. *Can Anesth Soc J*, **28**, 259–262.

Roila, F., Tonato, M., Basurto, C. (1988) Anti-emetic activity of high doses of metoclopramide in cisplatin treated cancer patients: a randomised double-blind trial of the Italian Oncology Group for Clinical Research. *J Clin Oncol*, **5**, 141–149.

Roila, F., Tonato, M., Basurto, C. *et al.* (1989) Protection from nausea and vomiting in cisplatin-treated patients: high-dose metoclopramide combined with methylprednisolone versus metoclopramide combined with dexamethasone and diphenhydramine: a study of the Italian Oncology Group for Clinical Research. *J Clin Oncol*, **7**(11), 1693–1700.

Roila, F., Tonato, M., Cognetti, F., *et al.* (1990) A double-blind, multi-centre, randomised, crossover study comparing the anti-emetic efficacy and tolerability of ondansetron vs ondansetron plus dexamethasone in cisplatin-treated patients. *Proc Am Soc Clin Oncol*, **9**, A1321.

Rowbotham, D.J. (1992) Current management of postoperative nausea and vomiting. *Br J Anaesth*, **69**, (Suppl. 1) 46S–59S.

Rowley, M.P. & Brown, T.C.K. (1982) Postoperative vomiting in children. *Anaesth Intens Care*, **10**, 309–313.

Rudd, J.A. & Naylor, R.J. (1990) Preliminary assessment of feverfew (*Tanecetum parthenium*) to antagonistic cisplatin-induced emesis in the ferret. *Br J Pharmacol*, **39**, 247P.

Ruff, P., Paska, W., Goedhals, L. *et al.* (1994) Ondansetron compared with granisetron in the prophylaxis of cisplatin-induced acute emesis: a multicentre double-blind, randomised, parallel-group study. *Oncology*, **51**, 113–118.

Russell, D. & Kenny, G.N.C. (1992) 5-HT$_3$ antagonists in postoperative nausea and vomiting. *Br J Anaesth*, **69**, (Suppl. 1) 63S–68S.

Sallan, S.E., Cronin, C., Zelen, M. & Zinberg, N.E. (1980) Antiemetics in patients receiving chemotherapy for cancer. *New Eng J Med*, **302**, 135–138.

Sampson, C. (1982) *The Neglected Ethic: Religious and Cultural Factors in the Care of Patients.* McGraw-Hill, London.

Santos, A. & Datta, S. (1984) Prophylactic use of droperidol for control of nausea and vomiting during spinal anaesthesia for caesarean section. *Anesth Analg*, **44**, 865.

Schwella, N., König, V., Schwerdtfeger, R. *et al.* (1994) Ondansetron for efficient control of emesis during total body irradiation. *Bone Marrow Transpl*, **13**, 169–171.

Schmoll, H-J. (1989) The role of ondansetron in the treatment of emesis induced by non-displatin-containing chemotherapy regimes. *Eur J Cancer Clin Oncol*, **25**, (Suppl. 1) S35–S49.

Scogna, D.M. & Smalley, R.V. (1979) Chemotherapy-induced nausea and vomiting. *Am J Nurs*, **79**, 1562–1564.

Scott, D.W., Donahue, D.C., Mastrovito, R.C. & Hakes, T.B. (1986)

Comparative trial of clinical relaxation and an antiemetic drug regimen in reducing chemotherapy-related nausea and vomiting. *Cancer Nursing*, **9**, 178–187.

Shah, Z.P. & Wilson, J. (1972) An evaluation of metoclopramide as an antiemetic in minor gynaecological surgery. *Br J Anaesth*, **44**, 865–867.

Shearer, E.S. & Hunter, J.M. (1992) Peri-operative fluid and electrolyte balance. *Current Anaesth Crit Care*, **3**, 71–76.

Simms, S.G., Rhodes, V.A. & Madsen, R.W. (1993) Comparison of prochlorperazine and lorazepam antiemetic regimens in the control of postchemotherapy symptoms. *Nurs Res*, **42**, 234–239.

Smessaert, A., Scher, C.A. & Artusio, J.F. (1959) Nausea and vomiting in the immediate postanesthetic period. *JAMA*, **170**, 2072–2076.

Smith, D.B., Newlands, E.S., Spruyt, O.W. *et al.* Ondansetron (GR38032F) plus dexamethasone: effective anti-emetic prophylaxis for patients receiving cytotoxic chemotherapy. *Br J Cancer*, **61**, 323–324.

Smith, I.E. (1990) A comparison of two dose levels of granisetron in patients receiving moderately emetogenic cytostatic chemotherapy. *Eur J Cancer*, **26**, (Suppl. 1) S19–S23.

Smyth, J.F., Coleman, R.E., Nicolson, M. *et al.* (1991) Does dexamethasone enhance the control of acute cisplatin induced emesis induced by ondansetron? *Br Med J*, **303**, 1423–1426.

Sorbe, B. & Berglind, A-M. (1992) Tropisetron, a new 5-HT$_3$ receptor antagonist, in the prevention of radiation-induced nausea, vomiting and diarrhoea. *Drugs*, **43**, (Suppl. 3) 33–39.

Soules, M.R., Hughes, C.L., Garcia, J.A., Livergood, C.H., Prystowsky, M.R. & Alexander, E. (1980) Nausea and vomiting of pregnancy: role of human chorionic gonadotrophin and 17-hydroxyprogesterone. *Obstet Gynaecol*, **55**, 696–700.

Spiess, J.L., Adelstein, D.J. & Hines, J.D. (1987) Evaluation of ethanol as an antiemetic in patients receiving cisplatin. *Clin Ther*, **9**, 400–404.

Stables, R., Andrews, P.L.R., Bailey, H.E. *et al.* (1987) Antiemetic properties of the 5-HT$_3$ receptor antagonist, GR38032F. *Cancer Treat Rev*, **14**, 333–336.

Steele, N., Gralla, R.J., Braun, D.W. & Young, C.W. (1980) Double blind comparison of the anti-emetic effects of nabilone and prochlorperazine on chemotherapy-induced emesis. *Cancer Treat Rep*, **64**, 219–224.

Stein, J.M. (1982) Factors affecting nausea and vomiting in the plastic surgery patient. *Plast Reconstr Surg*, **70**, 505–511.

Stott, J.R.R. (1986) Mechanisms and treatment of motion sickness. In *Nausea and Vomiting: Mechanisms and Treatment*. pp. 110–129. (eds: C.J. Davis, G.V. Lake-Bakaar & D.G. Grahame-Smith). Springer-Verlag, Berlin.

Strohl, R.A. (1988) The nursing role in radiation oncology: symptom management of acute and chronic reactions. *Oncol Nurs Forum*, **15**, 429–434.

Stunkard, A., Foster, G., Glassman, J. *et al.* (1985) Retrospective exaggeration of symptoms: vomiting after gastric surgery for obesity. *Psychosom Med*, **47**, 150–155.

Thomas, A.E. (1987) Pre-operative fasting – a question of routine? *Nursing Times*, **83**(49), 46–47.

Tisserand, R. (1988) *Aromatherapy for Everyone*. Penguin Health, West Drayton.

Tonato, M., Roila, F. & Del Favero, A. (1993) Nausea in anti-cancer treatment: measurement and mechanisms. In: *Emesis in Anti-cancer Therapy. Mechanisms and Treatment* (eds P.L.R. Andrews and G.J. Sanger). Chapman & Hall, London.

Tornetta, F.J. (1969) Clinical studies with the new antiemetic metoclopramide, *Anesth Analg*, **48**, 198–204.

Treasure, J., Schmidt, Troop, N., Tiller, J., Todd, G. & Keilen, M. (1994) First step in managing bulimia nervosa: controlled trial of therapeutic manual. *Br Med J.* **308**, 686–689.

Triozzi, P.L. & Laszlo, J. (1987) Optimum management of nausea and vomiting in cancer chemotherapy. *Drugs*, **34**, 136–149.

Troesch, L.M., Rodehaver, C.B., Delaney, E.A. & Yanes, B. (1993) The influence of guided imagery on chemotherapy-related nausea and vomiting. *Oncol Nurs Forum*, **20**, 1179–1185.

Turton, P. (1989) Touch me, feel me, heal me. *Nursing Times*, **85**, 19, 42–44.

Ummenhofer, W., Frei, F.J., Kern, C., Urwyler, A. & Drewe, J. (1993) Ondansetron reduces postoperative nausea and vomiting in children. *Anesthesiology*, **79**, (3A) A1192.

van der Walt, J.H., Jacob, R., Murrell, D. & Bentley, M. (1990) The perioperative effect of oral premedication in children. *Anaesth Int Care*, **18**, 5–10.

Vance, J.P., Neill, R.S. & Norris, W. (1973) The incidence and aetiology of postoperative nausea and vomiting in a plastic surgical unit. *Br J Plast Surg*, **26**, 226–339.

Van Thiez, D.H., Gavaler, J.S., Joshi, S.N. & Sara, R.K. (1977) Heartburn of pregnancy. *Gastroenterology*, **72**, 666–668.

Venner, P. (1990) Control of cisplatin-induced nausea and vomiting: a double-blind comparative study. SmithKline Beecham Satellite Symposium *15th International Cancer Congress*, Hamburg.

Wampler, G. (1983) The pharmacology and clinical effectiveness of phenothiazines and related drugs for managing chemotherapy-induced emesis. *Drugs*, **25**, (Suppl. 1) 35–51.

Wang, S.C. & Borison, H.L. (1950) The Vomiting Center: a critical experimental analysis. *Arch Neurol Psych*, **63**, 928–941.

Warrington, P.S., Allan, S.G., Cornbleet, M.A. *et al.* (1986) Optimising antiemesis in cancer chemotherapy: efficacy of continuous versus intermittent infusion of high dose metoclopramide in emesis induced by cisplatin. *Br Med J*, **293**, 1334–1335.

Webb, P. (1988) Teaching patients and relatives. In: *Oncology for Nurses and Health Care Professionals*, (series ed. R. Tiffany) 2nd ed, Vol. 2, Chapter 6, pp. 86–101. Chapman & Hall, London.

Webb, P. (1994) *Health Promotion and Patient Education. A Professional's Guide*, (ed. Patricia Webb). Chapman & Hall, London.

Weightman, W.M., Zacharias, M. & Herbison, P. (1987) Traditional Chinese acupuncture as an anti-emetic. *Br Med J*, **295**, 1379–1389.

Welch, D.A. (1980) Assessment of nausea and vomiting in cancer patients undergoing external beam radiotherapy. *Cancer Nursing*, **3**, 365–371.

White, P.F. & Schafer, A. (1987) Nausea and vomiting: causes and prophylaxis. *Semin Anesth*, **6**, 300–308.

Whitehead, S.A., Andrews, P.L.R. & Chamberlain, G.V.P. (1992) Characterisation of nausea and vomiting in early pregnancy: a survey of 1000 women. *J Obstet Gynaecol*, **12**, 364–369.

Wickham, R. (1989) Managing chemotherapy-related nausea and vomiting: the state of the art. *Oncol Nurs Forum*, **16**, 563–574.

Wilkinson, S. (1991) Factors which influence how nurses communicate with cancer patients. *J Adv Nurs*, **16**, 677–688.

Wilkinson, S.M. (1994) The changing pressures for cancer nursing 1986–1993. Submitted to *Eur J Cancer Care*.

Yamahara, J., Rong, H.Q., Naitoh, Y. *et al.* (1989a) Inhibition of cytotoxic drug-induced vomiting in sunctus by a ginger constituent. *J Ethnopharmacol*, **27**, 353–355.

Yamahara, J., Rong, H.Q., Iwamoto, M. *et al.* (1989b) Active component of ginger exhibiting anti-serotoninergic action. *Phytotherapy Res*, **3**, 70–71.

Yentis, S.M. & Bissonnette, B. (1992) Ineffectiveness of acupuncture and droperidol in preventing vomiting following stabismus repair in children. *Can J Anaesth*, **39**, 151–154.

Young, R.W. (1986) Mechanisms and treatment of radiation-induced nausea and vomiting. In: *Nausea and Vomiting: Mechanisms and Treatment*, pp. 94–109. (eds C.J. Davis, G.V. Lake-Bakaar, D.G. Grahame-Smith). Springer-Verlag, Berlin.

Zook, D.J. & Yasko, J.M. (1983) Psychological factors: their effect on nausea and vomiting experienced by clients receiving chemotherapy. *Oncol Nurs Forum*, **10**, 76–81.

Zoubek, A., Kronberger, M., Puschman, A. & Gadner, H. (1993) Ondansetron in the control of chemotherapy-induced and radiotherapy-induced emesis in children with malignancies. *Anti-cancer Drugs*, **4**, (Suppl.) 17–21.

APPENDIX A:
USEFUL ADDRESSES

Patient leaflets on diet, how to cope with nausea and vomiting and a variety of other topics are available from:

BACUP (British Association of Cancer United Patients): 3, Bath Place, Rivington Street, London EC2A 3JR.

CANCERLINK: 17, Britannia Street, London WC1X 9JN; 9 Castle Terrace, Edinburgh EH1 2DP.

The Royal Marsden Hospital: Fulham Road, London SW3 6JJ. Contact Mrs V. Speechley

Other useful addresses are as follows:

Breast Cancer and Mastectomy Association: 15/19 Britten Street, London SW3 3TZ. Tel. 0171 867 8275.

British Colostomy Association: 15 Station Road, Reading, Berks RG1 1LG. Tel. 01734 391537.

The Stoma Advisory Service: Hollister Ltd, Rectory Court, 42 Broad Street, Wokingham, Berks RG11 1AB. Tel. 01800 521377.

National Association of Laryngectomee Clubs: Ground Floor, 6 Rickett Street, Fulham, London SW6 1RU. Tel. 0171 381 9993.

APPENDIX B: ANSWERS TO SELF ASSESSMENT QUESTIONS

Chapter 2

1. (a) F	2. (a) T	3. (a) T	4. (a) T
(b) T	(b) F	(c) T	(b) F
(c) F	(c) T	(c) F	(c) T
(d) T	(d) T	(d) F	(d) F
			(e) T

5. (a) T	6. (a) F	7. (a) T	8. (a) T
(b) F	(b) T	(b) F	(b) T
(c) F	(c) T	(c) T	(c) T
	(d) T	(d) F	(d) T
	(e) F		

9. (a) T
   (b) F
   (c) T

Chapter 3

1. (a) T	2. (a) T	3. (a) T	4. (a) T
(b) F	(b) F	(b) T	(b) F
(c) T	(c) F	(c) F	(c) T
(d) F		(d) T	(d) F

5. (a) F	6. a should	7. a and c	8. (a) T
(b) F	be ticked	should be	(b) F
(c) T		ticked	(c) F
(d) F			(d) T
(e) F			(e) F

9. (a) 3	10. (a) F	11. (a) T
(b) 1	(b) F	(b) F
(c) 2	(c) T	(c) F
(d) 4		

12. (a) F	13. (a) T	14. a and c	15. (a) 4
(b) T	(b) F	should	(b) 1
(c) F	(c) T	be ticked	(c) 3
(d) F	(d) F		(d) 2

16. (a) T	17. (a) T
(b) T	(b) F
(c) F	(c) F
(d) T	(d) T
(e) F	

Chapter 4

1. (a) T	2. (a) F	3. (a) T	4. A – 6
(b) F	(b) F	(b) F	B – 4,5,6
(c) T	(c) T	(c) T	C – 1,2,4
(d) F	(d) F	(d) T	D – 3
(e) T		(e) T	
(f) F			

5. (a) T	6. b and e	7. (a) T	8. (a) T
(b) T	should be	(b) T	(b) T
(c) T	ticked	(c) F	(c) F
(d) T			(d) T

9. (a) F	10. (a) F	11. (a) T
(b) F	(b) T	(b) F
(c) T	(c) T	(c) F
	(d) F	(d) T

12. a and b	13. (a) T	14. (a) F	15. (a) T
should be	(b) T	(b) F	(b) T
ticked	(c) F	(c) F	(c) F
	(d) T	(d) F	(d) F

Chapter 5

1. (a) F	2. (a) F	3. (a) F	4. (a) F
(b) T	(b) T	(b) T	(b) F
(c) T	(c) F	(c) T	(c) F
	(d) F	(d) T	(d) F

5. (a) F
(b) F
(c) F
(d) T

Chapter 6

1. (a) F
   (b) F
   (c) F

2. (a) T
   (b) T
   (c) T
   (d) T

3. (a) T
   (b) F
   (c) F

4. (a) F
   (b) F
   (c) F
   (d) F
   (e) T

5. (a) T
   (b) F
   (c) F
   (d) F

INDEX